Marketing Your Hospital

A Strategy for Survival

Norman H. McMillan

AHA

American Hospital Publishing, Inc.,
a wholly owned subsidiary
of the American Hospital Association

Library of Congress Cataloging in Publication Data

McMillan, Norman H., 1925-
    Marketing your hospital.

    "AHA catalog no. 136100."
    Bibliography: p.
    1. Hospitals—Marketing.   2. Public relations—
Hospitals.   I. Title.
RA965.5.M37   1984   362.1'1'0688   84-21576
ISBN 0-939450-51-8

AHA is a service mark of American Hospital Association
used under license by American Hospital Publishing, Inc.

Frank Sabatino, Editor
Marjorie E. Weissman, Manager, Book Editorial Department
Dorothy Saxner, Vice-President, Books

Cover art courtesy of Ted Peterson Associates, Hinsdale, Illinois

To Benny . . . and one more time, for Marge

Contents

PART 4 Market Positioning and Impression Statements

PART 5 Marketing to Doctors

PART 6 Public Relations

PART 7 Design and Graphics

PART 8 Advertising

PART **9** The Marketing Budget and the Marketing Audit

PART **10** Epilog

Foreword

In his book *Planning for Survival: A Handbook for Hospital Trustees,* published by the American Hospital Association in 1978, Norman H. McMillan called upon hospital trustees, administrators, and medical staffs to adopt business techniques for the long-range planning of health care facilities. In *Marketing Your Hospital: A Strategy for Survival,* he urges that same audience to apply equally successful business techniques to market their services to health care consumers.

Mr. McMillan has an extensive background in marketing and advertising for the corporate world and more than 20 years of experience as a hospital trustee. Now a corporate officer of Montgomery Ward & Company, Chicago, Mr. McMillan has held the positions of senior vice-president of plans and marketing for the advertising agency N. W. Ayer & Son, and president of marketing and strategic planning for CBS Specialty Stores, a division of CBS, Inc. He has also served as chairman of the board of trustees of St. Mary's Rehabilitation Center, Minneapolis, and as a member of the board of governors of Methodist Hospital, Minneapolis.

Introduction

This book is about marketing and health care. It is long on the practice of marketing, long on making it work. It is not a book on theoretical concepts.

At the time I began to write this book, I was convinced that hospitals needed to get acquainted with marketing and that society, not to mention hospitals, would be the beneficiary. That conviction remains intact and has strengthened as a result of working on specific health care marketing projects and helping to get a number of hospitals organized for the age of marketing. It has survived the challenge of a few hundred conversations with trustees, chief executive officers, and physicians.

But as these people have challenged me and the marketing ideas I advocate, I have changed my views. I now believe that there is more marketing activity in our hospitals than is generally recognized in the health care industry. Although many doctors and trustees are still unused to the notion of a hospital using advertising, many hospitals already are using this major marketing tool to present annual reports to the community and for specific programs. In my opinion, the efforts often are inept, but the fact is that many hospitals are already using advertising successfully.

I also find much solid marketing work going on in some very surprising places within hospitals, for instance, in the chaplain's office and in social workers' offices.

Finally, the public relations functions, which always were the obvious outposts of marketing in hospitals, are winning increasing support from both the CEO and the board of trustees. This has come about as hospitals, under pressure, became aware that they are legitimate targets of interest for the media. At the moment, however, their marketing efforts tend to be random and accidental.

In many hospitals, attitude has emerged as the biggest problem. As I talk with the trustees and CEOs around the country, it seems to me that the bigger the hospital, the bigger the problem is. I know of one 60-bed hospital that does a superb marketing job, and yet I know of a 1,200-bed multihospital system that is doing a poor job, in spite of the fact that it pours much time and many resources into marketing.

A theory emerges: Administrators and trustees of small hospitals are close to the action, close to the customers. They develop marketing talent in response to the need. As hospitals get bigger, there are more layers and greater distances between top management and "the market." Big hospitals talk the best fight, but small hospitals sometimes perform best.

The best news, however, is probably just this: Most of our hospitals already have a fair amount of marketing activity going on. We just need to organize it, supplement it, and give it good management direction. This book explains how.

1 The Case for Marketing Your Hospital

Marketing Defined

What is marketing? A modest definition, but one that says it all, is this:
- Find out what people want, and give them more of it
- Find out what people don't want, and give them less of it

The definition is simple enough, and it
- Implies a willingness to spend money to find out what consumers think about the health care they get at your hospital and at its competitors
- Suggests that you will do this methodically, objectively, and professionally and not rely on your own acquaintances, patients, or family, because they are not typical
- Suggests that you respect your customers as individuals, not just the money they represent to you personally or to your hospital
- Means an openness, a willingness to communicate, and a desire to put the facts on the table, even if the facts are not as appealing as you might wish
- Says that when you have a legitimate cause, you are entitled to communicate it to your constituents and attempt to persuade them that your views are important and valid
- Suggests a willingness on your part to communicate with any legitimate newsperson at any time about any subject, unless that communication breaks a law or violates the right to privacy of a patient or an employee
- Suggests that you will use the same cost-effective, low-cost communication media that professionals employ—newspapers, radio, TV, magazines
- Means you will not hesitate to use the mass media because of old-fashioned notions about mass media being unprofessional, unseemly, or undignified

Marketing means all of these things.

Marketing Is Not a Four-Letter Word

Marketing is not a four-letter word, something bad, negative, unprofessional, or beneath our dignity. It is a battery of proven, 40-year old techniques for listening and learning, speaking and persuading, teaching and communicating.

Many persons who populate hospital boards of trustees, hospital managements, and medical staffs start with a prejudice. They think marketing is beneath their dignity. They use words and phrases like "professional standards," "ethical conduct," or "gentlemanly behavior" to justify their prejudice and delay the use of well-proven marketing tools. Without bothering to understand what marketing is all about, they put it down. What a shame!

On one occasion, after giving a talk to the medical staff of a hospital and their spouses, I was verbally attacked by a doctor's wife. The words came pouring out:

- How dare you equate the practice of medicine to business . . .
- You commercial people are trying to interfere with the sacred trust that exists between a doctor and the patient . . .
- My husband studied for twelve years so he could tell patients . . .
- You owe the doctors an apology for suggesting they need to listen to consumers: society should be listening to them . . .

This woman probably speaks for many in health care. That's the prejudice about marketing.

It is not a sin to listen. It is not a sin to communicate. Marketing is okay; marketing is positive. It is good for consumers and good for your hospital because it brings the two together. Marketing is not a four-letter word.

Hospitals Are out of Touch

An article that appeared in February 1980 in the *San Francisco Chronicle* (reprinted below and through page 8) is representative of perhaps a hundred other articles you have seen that attack hospitals, doctors, or the whole health care system. The article says that society and the health care system are out of touch with each other and are not communicating. There is a lot of confrontation, a lot of finger-pointing, a lot of headline-making, and not much communication.

Marketing can help put society and hospitals back on speaking terms by bringing the two together again. Converting your hospital into a consumer-oriented marketing enterprise is urgent business. Among other things, it will result in making articles like the one quoted much less newsworthy to the media.

COST-CUTTING MEASURES
Revolution in Health Care Is Proposed*

By Charles Petit
Science Correspondent

A massive plan to turn the priorities of health care in California upside down—emphasizing improved environment and living habits over doctor and hospital care—is being proposed by state health planners, who are faced with the soaring cost of conventional, high-technology medicine.

If adopted—and if written into law and regulation—the plan might mean widescale closures and mergers of hospitals, strict guidelines telling doctors what specialties they might practice and how they would get paid, and ambitious attempts to get people to

*© *San Francisco Chronicle*, 1980. Reprinted by permission.

change their ways—including eating, exercise, and smoking habits.

The plan, described in a main volume and extensive appendixes, is certain to cause controversy. Critics, especially those in the hospital industry, have already attacked it, but health planning agencies generally welcome its ambitious attempt to bring order to the state's multibillion-dollar health care system.

The product of several years of effort by a 17-person staff at the Office of Statewide Health Planning and Development in Sacramento, aided by 98 consultants and advisory committee members, the "California Health Plan, 1980-1985" is now the subject of public hearings throughout the state.

In San Francisco, there will be two hearings tomorrow, at 2 p.m. and at 7 p.m. in Conference Room 1, Building A, Fort Mason at Bay and Franklin streets.

Henry Zeretsky, director of the state agency that produced the proposal, said the plan "challenges the entrenched position of 100 years of health care, that is that health is the prerogative of the physicians and hospitals. We're not saying doctors are dangerous to your health, but they're not the last word either."

Human behavior, biology, and environment are put by the plan as more important to health than large-scale use of doctors and hospitals.

In line with the growing "holistic" or "humanistic" health movements, the plan defines health as "a state of complete physical, mental, and social well-being and not merely the absence of disease or infirmity."

Suggested ways to maintain and improve the health of the state's residents—supposedly at an affordable price—include encouraging more fluoridation of water, tax incentives for corporations to provide gymnasiums and exercise facilities for employees, greatly increased nutrition and health education in schools, tighter anti-pollution enforcement, elimination of sugar-rich vending machine foods in public buildings, and general "promotion of health and prevention of disease."

The bulk of the hefty proposal, however, deals more with putting a lid on the cost of conventional medical care than promotion of healthy lifestyles.

The strategy may face tough going in Sacramento, where lawmakers have in recent weeks turned down several attempts to put tough shackles on hospital expansion and rate increases.

The plan nonetheless outlines a broad attack on how hospitals and doctors are paid, where they are located, and what they do. Of the 600 hospitals in the state now, Zeretsky said, "We could pick out 210 hospitals in California that nobody would miss, and by eliminating them save $700 million to $1 billion."

To change what is perceived as a serious overconcentration of highly paid specialists in major cities, while there are too few "primary care" physicians such as family practice doctors throughout the state, the plan suggests various "economic incentives" to control where doctors live and what services they offer.

"If rationalized economic incentives fail to moderate growth (of concentrations of highly paid specialists), more direct controls may be required," the plan says. To doctors who already feel hemmed in by growing regulation of medical care, this raises the specter of government agencies determining where a doctor may practice in order to get reimbursement from government health plans.

High on its list of priorities is elimination of the way state and federal health insurance programs, such as Medicare and Medi-Cal, now pay doctors and hospitals.

As an alternative, the plan—in line with current Brown administration policy—encourages creation of health maintenance organizations, or HMOs. In HMOs—the big Kaiser health plan is the prime example—physicians are paid salaries. The intent is for the organization to make the most money by keeping its patients as healthy as possible with the least use of costly hospitalization and medical procedures.

The plan has, inevitably, drawn sharp fire from the established health industry. Charles White, director of research for the California Hospital Association, said, "It isn't a plan; it just states a bunch of hostile policy beliefs and opinions. It talks grandly about changing people's behavior and making them more healthy, but then it falls back on the same old tired accusations about the medical care systems, attacking doctors, hospitals, and high technology and calling everybody a crook."

Redressing the Balance

The case for the use of marketing techniques by hospitals is a straight-forward one and is founded on this bedrock:

- Hospitals are here to serve consumers' needs. The mission of the hospital within its community is to help patients get well and stay well. Consumers are a hospital's reason for existence.
- Consumers have a legitimate interest in hospitals and what goes on there. Measuring and understanding their concerns are legitimate and urgent actions.
- Consumers in total—that is, *society*—will express their concerns through legislation when either costs or concerns get high enough.
- Hospitals that do not listen well or interact effectively will probably fail or be penalized for unresponsiveness to consumer needs.
- Hospitals that can both listen and communicate effectively will thrive.

That is the case for marketing. Is it important? Yes, because it is how you and your hospital, and ultimately the whole health care system, will redress the balance. It is how hospitals, frequently suspect and under a cloud, will earn the right once again to represent consumers and to deal with them without as much outside intervention as there is now.

Marketing will allow hospitals to enter and win a race with the politicians to see who can be the most effective advocate for consumer interests. And *that* is good news for consumers.

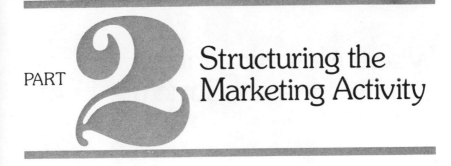

PART **2** Structuring the Marketing Activity

Where Marketing Fits into the Hospital Structure

Many plans and programs are put together in hospitals every year, and the work is done confidently and efficiently because the subject generally fits comfortably within the range of the hospital's competence. Now, along comes another discipline—marketing—and, if your hospital is like most, marketing causes:

- Disbelief that the hospital is even contemplating the use of marketing techniques
- Some doubt that marketing is "real," as a result of a lack of knowledge of what it is all about
- Anxiety about how marketing might influence existing activities and departments

So here in diagram form is where marketing fits among a hospital's activities.

LONG-RANGE PLAN	
MARKETING PLAN	FINANCIAL PLAN

The diagram shows that the marketing plan should be thought of as the twin of the familiar financial plan, neither subservient nor superior, but equal. Both are controlled by the hospital's long-range plan. Both work toward long-range objectives, and neither has an independent life.

The key point is that marketing exists to help the hospital achieve its long-range plans as well as solve some of its immediate problems. With that simple idea established, we now move to an examination of the marketing hierarchy.

Marketing encompasses a diverse group of activities, each of which is represented by a specialist who tends to think of his particular piece of the pie as just a little more important than the other pieces. This makes for confusion until it is sorted out.

Another diagram may be helpful.

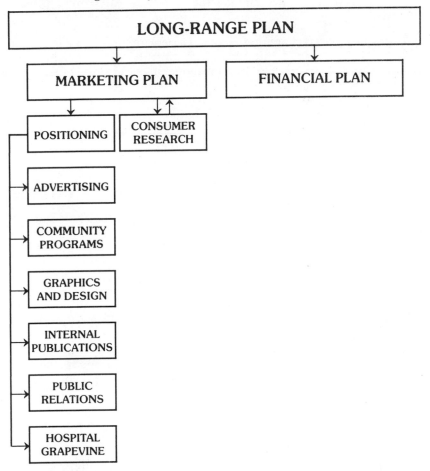

This diagram is an extension of the first one and covers three additional aspects of marketing.

- It shows the pivotal role of consumer research in a "business" organized to service consumers. It is used up front to listen with, and it is used after programs have been implemented to assess their effectiveness. It can also be used to learn from the physicians and others on the hospital medical staff.
- The diagram introduces a new word, *positioning,* as the extension of the marketing plan. Positioning is the one idea that all phases of a marketing plan are expected to support and develop. Positioning is what the hospital has decided it wants to be known for.
- The marketing plan provides direction for all of the marketing

elements, none of which is unrelated or independent. The marketing director of a hospital uses the plan to organize the efforts of each activity.

The two previous diagrams establish a pecking order, or a list of the priorities of marketing. But most important, the diagrams show the relationship of marketing to the long-range plan and to the much more familiar financial plan.

The simplest kind of definition of what marketing is all about in the hospital is shown in the following diagram.

LISTEN ←→ TALK	
TALK ←→ LISTEN	

The diagram indicates that marketing demands that you learn to listen responsibly to the market. That means an organized sampling of consumer opinions on a steady basis. It means much more than just good listening to the complaints that come to your attention, or the monitoring of what is being said in the hospital, because all of this listening is heavily biased. Listening also extends to occasional projects to ensure that you are hearing your physicians, nurses, and employees accurately.

The diagram also implies that you will develop your skills and your willingness to communicate forthrightly to all the persons who are interested in the hospital and in a way that fills their needs. In other words, before you start "transmitting," figure out what it is you want to say.

Marketing Strategy for Hospitals

Hospitals need a marketing strategy for dealing with the public, just as businesses do and for exactly the same reason: to ensure that their many marketing activities are coordinated and that their staffs are working toward the same common goals.

Many hospitals today suffer from the same malady most businesses suffered from some years ago: they never seem to be able to get it all together. They never get all of the functions, all of the troops, headed in the same direction. Each activity appears to lead an independent life, depending almost solely on the chief executive officer to knock heads and keep them all coordinated. And, of course, the CEO has many other things to worry about. The result is much frustration, poor communication, and much less than optimum performance. What those hospitals need is a strategy for dealing with the public.

The marketing strategy controls and gives specific focus to many functions, including:

- The activities of the public relations director
- Internal newsletters and the hospital's house organ
- The annual report
- Graphics such as external and internal signs, logotypes, and symbols
- The appearance and ambience of all public places in the hospital
- The language, content, and appearance of all printed material given to patients (with a particular view to converting all communication from hospitalese to plain English)
- Public relations and contacts with news reporters
- The use of media advertising
- Consumer research to feed the marketing process and bring the hospital into harmony with public needs and desires
- Support for the fund-raising effort (but *not* fund raising)

Every facet of the hospital's activities that touches the public needs coordination and consistency. The many voices of the hospital, all of which contribute to forming the public's opinion of the hospital, need direction. Otherwise, meaningless noise, not a harmonious chorus, is the result. What makes the difference is the presence of a marketing strategy laid down formally in an annual marketing plan.

Outline of the Annual Marketing Plan

You do not need to follow a rigid format as you pull the marketing strategy together. However, you have to start somewhere, so here is the time-tested outline that most marketing people would subscribe to, adapted to hospital use for an annual marketing plan:

I. Situation
II. Mission Statement
III. Marketing Objectives
IV. Target Audience(s)
    A. Consumers
    B. Doctors/nurses
    C. Donors
V. Market Positioning/Impression Statement
VI. Annual Recommendations
    A. Research
        1. To measure performance of the marketing activity
        2. To develop data for decision making
    B. Public relations activities
    C. Media advertising
    D. Internal communications
        1. Patient
        2. Staff
    E. Design and graphics
    F. Budget

Now some elaboration on the outline.

Item I, Situation, refers to a backgrounding section in which the marketing director describes what has occurred at the hospital (or in the community) in the previous year that affects the marketing effort. This is an introductory section. Get the key facts described, but keep it brief.

Item II, Mission Statement, is a simple pickup of the hospital's mission statement. It should prove to be the main fountainhead of influence on the marketing strategy. However, in most hospitals (about 95 percent), it will prove to be fairly innocuous and therefore not helpful. The marketing plan should provide an interpretation of the mission statement that yields more direction.*

Item III, Marketing Objectives, should state the objectives of the marketing effort and numerically weight them, that is, assign the importance attached to each objective. The objectives should be stated in such a way that performance can be measured at the end of the year.

Item IV, Target Audience, means precisely who you are trying to reach with the marketing effort, for example, "adult consumers between the ages of 25 and 40 with at least two years of college who reside within five miles of the hospital." Another target audience might be "all physicians in the metropolitan area who are not on our medical staff." The establishment of a target audience requires that choices be made. Do not settle for such vague descriptions as "all consumers," or "all potential donors."

Item V, Impression Statement and Market Positioning, are so important that all of part 4 of this book is dedicated to them. Having selected the audience(s) to be reached, you must decide what you want to communicate or, more precisely, what it is you want your audiences to remember. This is the impression statement. It should be a couple of paragraphs long, but no more than a half page, and it is probably the most important direction the plan will provide. It is therefore to be worded with great care, and it is worth effort. The statement will influence all aspects of your marketing effort. (This subject is discussed in detail in part 4.)

Item VI, Annual Recommendations, expresses your plan, how you are going to accomplish the objectives, how you will "land" the message implied by your impression statement in the heads of those who populate your target audiences. The plan should include specific recommendations for each of the functional areas indicated in the outline (research, public relations, and so forth). This is the general outline of the annual marketing plan. It describes the territory you must cover, but you need not follow it slavishly.

Now we want to turn to the heart of the marketing activity: how you should go about developing your marketing research to establish your market positioning.

---

*See McMillan, N. H. *Planning for Survival: A Handbook for Hospital Trustees.* Chicago: American Hospital Association, 1978.

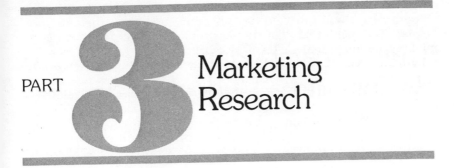

PART **3** Marketing
Research

The Research Plan Begins with a Budget

How much should your consumer research budget be? A large hospital, with staff expertise to use consumer data, could intelligently spend $200,000 annually in the pursuit of knowledge about consumer attitudes. However, that is not the way for most hospitals to begin, because most are not ready to use the data that such an outlay on consumer research could provide. In most hospitals it will make more sense to start small and increase the budget as the hospital's ability to use the data productively grows.

Here is a starting point for thinking about your consumer research budget: you should spend about 0.5 percent of your hospital's annual budget on consumer research. Using that figure as a guide, and depending on the size of your hospital's budget, research outlays would look like this:

Total Hospital Budget	Annual Consumer Research Budget at 0.5%
$ 3,000,000	$ 15,000
$ 5,000,000	$ 25,000
$10,000,000	$ 50,000
$20,000,000	$100,000
$50,000,000	$250,000

The bare-bones minimum research budget is $15,000, even for a small hospital. With a budget greater than $250,000, the research that additional dollars could buy becomes marginal, even for a large hospital.

The cost of knowledge is high, but the cost of ignorance about consumers in a hospital's trade area is much higher, as many hospitals have proven in the past several years. Budgets of the size proposed should buy important insights about how consumers view hospitals.

The Key Is Spending Smart, Not Big

In consumer research, the key is to spend smart, not big. It is relatively easy to spend a large amount of money, but it is relatively difficult to get high productivity at low cost. That is particularly true in the case of hospitals because most do not have a staff of experienced marketing people who know how to develop and interpret market data and then put them to use.

The abilities to generate and use data must be developed together. For that reason we generally counsel spending judiciously in the beginning, on well-defined projects, so that the management, physicians, and board members can learn to use this tool.

As part of the program to "spend smart" you should remember that the purpose of the hospital's marketing research is to develop original data—proprietary information that cannot be looked up in a book or a standard reference. Therefore, you should first make sure that the data you want are not already freely available. A good place to begin your search is in computerized bibliographies, access to which is usually available for a modest fee. Some sources are the American Hospital Association, the Department of Health and Human Services, and many universities Also, many health systems agencies have developed market data that will be useful.

In the end, however, spending smart will mean that your consumer research program is as carefully planned as you can make it.

Here is the outline we recommend for the research plan:

A. Purpose of the consumer research
B. Objectives
C. Specific programs, including:
   1. Who will be in charge
   2. How this research might be significant
D. Who will review results of the research program and develop recommendations

On the basis of this outline, here is how the consumer research plan of a hypothetical 250-bed city hospital with a $12 million budget might look:

Consumer Research Plan for Loving Arms Hospital

A. Purpose

The purpose of the research plan is to provide data about consumer attitudes on issues facing the hospital. The results will be used to help the management and the trustees in their marketing and long-range planning decisions.

B. Objectives

1. Determine consumers' perceptions of Loving Arms Hospital relative to its three principal competitors on the west side of the city. In particular, consumer perceptions of the major strengths and weaknesses of each of the four hospitals will be developed. This specifically will include ratings of the major medical departments of each hospital.

2. Determine consumers' perceptions of the alternative programs that the board of trustees is now considering, including:
   - Upgrading the hospital's current facilities to place 30 percent of beds in single rooms
   - Converting rooms in B wing to nursing home facilities
   - Establishing a new drug abuse treatment center

3. Develop a performance monitoring system so that, at yearly intervals, various services of the hospital can be measured relative to other hospitals.

4. Develop a system of review and actions to ensure that the hospital benefits from the results of the research program.

C. Programs

Total cost of the programs is $81,000, allocated as follows:

1. Competitive strength survey
   Requested by W. Grimes, chairman, Long-Range Planning Committee
   Due date: 6/20
   Cost: $23,700
   This research will produce statistically projectable data for households in Loving Arms' service area, including data on patients who use other hospitals.

2. First annual performance monitor
   Requested by E. Benson, CEO
   Due date: 7/10
   Cost: $19,200
   Our hospital is here to serve consumers. The purpose of this study is to measure our performance as viewed by consumers, including families who have been to the hospital as patients or visitors and those who have not, but who have opinions about

the hospital. We will measure perceptions of nonmedical factors such as:

- Parking
- Food service
- Emergency department service
- Effectiveness of the staff in consumer communication
- Business office procedures
- Other

Data will lead to corrective action programs, and results will be monitored annually.

3. General health issues
Requested by the Council of Hospitals
Due date: 7/10
Cost: $2,750
All hospitals in the community have joined together to gather information of general use that will be used to develop information on the health system agency's proposals. It will be offered to the HSA and the media. Our share of the study is $2,750.

4. Survey of medical staff
Requested by E. Benson, CEO
Due date: 7/10
Cost: $16,600
To determine the attitudes about our hospital compared to other hospitals, data should disclose our shortcomings, strengths, and risks. The survey also should include a sample of doctors practicing in the service area who are not on this hospital's medical staff.

5. Nursing study
Requested by W. Grimes, chairman, Long-Range Planning Committee
Due date: 9/10
Cost: $7,750
To learn why nurses who are attracted to the hospital do not come to work here and why nurses leave, the survey should cover applicants, new graduates, and nurses who resign. Data will help recruit and retain nurses.

6. Special projects
Requested as needed
Due date: undetermined
Cost: $11,000
This budget is reserved for special projects that are expected to be generated out of the first research phases. Projects will be subject to the approval of E. Benson, CEO.

D. Review
All consumer research will be reviewed first by the marketing

director and then presented to the CEO. It will be the responsibility of the marketing director to ensure that all research findings are communicated to all affected management staff.

It is also understood in this first year that management and trustees will need to develop the capability to use data productively and act on findings. Making sure that the information is properly used and acted on will be the responsibility of the marketing director.

Hire a Pro

Your hospital cannot afford bad data; they may be even worse than no data. Obtaining accurate measurements of public opinion is a job for the best professional you can find. Do not underestimate the difficulty of the job or the degree of professionalism needed.

Politicians and companies that sell consumer products, whose livelihoods rest on reliable assessments of consumer attitudes, do not make that mistake. They are not amateurs, nor should you be when it comes to measuring public opinion. Highly trained professionals on their staffs hire other professionals in independent research firms.

Unless you propose hiring an adequate staff of market research professionals when you embark on your research effort, the best thing to do is to find a competent research company. Here are some guidelines for finding the best firm for your purposes:

- Get recommendations from people who work for firms that sell consumer products or services.
- Screen at least three research firms. Look at their client lists. Are the clients well known to you? Can you check references? Bigger is not always better, yet the presence of big clients usually denotes a high level of sophistication. Look for the kinds of work they are doing and the problems they have been solving for clients.
- Look for a company that has worked in the health field. If possible, find one that has recent experience with hospitals—the more of each the better. Such a company may be difficult to find, because few hospitals have yet become involved in consumer research. This is easily the most important criterion.
- Look at the qualifications and experience of the staff professionals, the professionals who will design the project, structure the questionnaire, and interpret the results. Don't get involved with the persons at the technical level who do the actual field work.
- Carefully consider the suggestion that you seek help from a local college or university. This suggestion is attractive to hospital managers because dealing with academia feels more comfortable and

less "commercial." If you deal with the universities, you may sometimes find that the project will cost you more and take longer than when you work with a commercial firm. In the real world, where hospital CEOs and trustees live, resources are limited and you will almost always be better off "going commercial."

- Once you have found a firm you have confidence in, stick with it. Your budget is too small, your time is too limited, and your personal expertise is too small for you to have different firms bid on the projects.

The message is "hire a pro," someone who has the experience and credentials to help your hospital. You should not spend your budget to help researchers learn about hospitals.

Getting into Specifics: Learning to Read Data

Consumer research may be a subject that is best illustrated by working through several sequences of research findings. Therefore, in this chapter and the four chapters that follow you will get a feel for consumer research by examining the responses of U.S. households to actual survey questions about health care.

In these chapters on consumer research, you will proceed from the general to the specific. In this chapter, you will focus on very general questions to show where consumers' heads have been in recent years concerning health care. In later chapters, you will examine specific questions that allow researchers to determine consumers' reaction to government intervention in health care delivery, to measure changes in consumers' attitudes, to provide background on competition, and to measure the attitudes of doctors and nurses.

The questions and answers displayed in this chapter are from a 1980 national survey of 455 U.S. households.*

Do you think that all persons should have equal medical care whether or not they can afford personally to pay for it?
Yes 77%
No. 11%
Not sure. 12%
The research shows that medical care is seen as a basic right by a large majority of consumers.

Do you believe that efforts by the government to regulate how much doctors can charge will reduce the cost of medical care?
Yes 45%
No. 43%
Not answering 12%

---

*Survey data presented in this chapter and other chapters in Part 3 were provided by Leo J. Shapiro and Associates, Inc., Chicago.

Consumers believe that government regulation of doctors' fees will be effective in lowering costs.

Are you in favor of or opposed to government regulation of doctors' fees?
In favor 55%
Opposed 34%
Not answering 11%
The data show strong support for government regulation of doctors' fees.

Are you in favor of or opposed to the government setting up and enforcing standards for the quality of medical care?
In favor 70%
Opposed 24%
Not answering 6%
Consumers express confidence in the government setting up and enforcing standards for the quality of medical care.

This research was completed several years ago. It is interesting to recall this period, when about 90 percent of trustees, doctors, and hospital administrators were saying, "It won't happen here." Consumers thought differently; the politicians heard this message and swung into action.

It is possible that the world of health care would be different today had it paid attention to consumer data like these. Maybe the health care industry could have changed the message, adjusted to it, or even have assumed a leadership role in changes arising from it.

More Specifics, More Questions and Answers

You will recall that a few years ago a government study startled many consumers because it claimed that doctors were performing many unneeded surgical procedures. Here are data from a study of 421 U.S. households conducted in 1976 that relate to this government report.

A recent study made by the government found that last year doctors performed more than two million surgeries that were not needed by patients. Did you happen to hear or read about this?
Yes 76%
No..................... 23%
Not answering 1%
These data show that an amazing number of consumers had read or heard about the government's allegations.

Assuming this figure is correct, are you inclined to feel that the figure is about normal or that it means something has gone wrong with American medical practice?
It means something has
gone wrong............ 62%
Figure is about normal 22%
No answer.............. 16%
The answer to this follow-up question indicates high agreement with the statement that something has gone wrong with U.S. medical practice.

A recent government study found that more than two million surgeries that were not needed by patients were performed last year. Do you think that the number of unnecessary operations and hospital admissions would go down if the government made an effort to control the quality of medical care?
Yes, the number would go
down 65%
No, number would not go
down 25%
No answer.............. 10%

Here, the majority of consumers agree that if the government became involved, unnecessary operations would decrease and admissions would decrease.

These data are static; they provide a glimpse of what consumers believe, or of their perceptions, at a particular time. But consumer perceptions are forever changing, and the data are most useful when both the direction and the amount of change are captured. This is illustrated in the next chapter.

Measuring the Change in Consumers' Attitudes

In the following examples, consumers rate the performance of various groups concerned with health. The example shows how consumer attitudes changed during a six-month interval in 1975 from February (255 respondents) to August (475 respondents), which is why your hospital should continuously measure and watch for shifts of opinion.

Overall, how good a job is being done by doctors and hospitals in providing adequate health service at a reasonable cost?

	Doctor			Hospitals		
	Feb.	**Aug.**	**Change**	**Feb.**	**Aug.**	**Change**
Excellent or good	**60%**	**44%**	**−16%**	**52%**	**36%**	**−16%**
Excellent	8%	11%		12%	8%	
Good	52%	33%		40%	28%	
Fair or poor	**39%**	**52%**	**+13%**	**45%**	**58%**	**+13%**
Fair	24%	30%		25%	30%	
Poor	15%	22%		20%	28%	
No answer	**1%**	**3%**	**+ 2%**	**3%**	**6%**	**+ 3%**

Overall, how good a job is being done by pharmaceutical companies and by the American Medical Association in providing adequate health service at a reasonable cost?

	Pharmaceutical Companies			American Medical Association		
	Feb.	**Aug.**	**Change**	**Feb.**	**Aug.**	**Change**
Excellent or good	**45%**	**34%**	**−11%**	**39%**	**30%**	**− 9%**
Excellent	10%	6%		5%	5%	
Good	35%	28%		34%	25%	
Fair or poor	**45%**	**58%**	**+13%**	**42%**	**55%**	**+13%**
Fair	25%	33%		24%	33%	
Poor	20%	25%		18%	22%	
No answer	**10%**	**8%**	**− 2%**	**19%**	**15%**	**− 4%**

Hospital managers who know what consumers are thinking about their hospital at any given time have an advantage, but the manager who knows where consumers are headed—that is, who understands the trends—has the capacity to dramatically outperform his hospital's competitor.

Research to Support the Marketing Effort

The previous examples of consumer research are broad. Now let's get more specific. The following examples, drawn from a consumer survey of 198 subjects conducted in 1977 in Minneapolis-St. Paul, show the kinds of data that an individual hospital is likely to need for either planning or marketing purposes.

What are some of the hospitals in this area that you know of?
Know of one or more
   hospitals 99%
Do not know of hospitals
   in area 1%
Average number of names
   given................... 2.4

If someone in your family had to be admitted to a hospital, do you know which one you would want to go to?
Yes 93%
No...................... 7%

Which hospital are you aware of? Would you prefer to go to that one?

	Aware of Hospital	Prefer the Hospital	Ratio
Hospital A	22.2%	19.7%	89%
Hospital B	18.7%	15.2%	81%
Hospital C	19.2%	12.1%	63%
Hospital D	10.6%	6.5%	61%
Hospital E	15.2%	9.1%	60%
Hospital F	25.8%	13.2%	51%
Hospital G	4.5%	1.5%	33%
Hospital H	13.1%	4.0%	31%

Working with a marketing person, a researcher developed a useful method of analysis to examine the strength of each individual hospital.

They looked at simple awareness and at preference, and then worked these two figures into a ratio that represents the percentage of persons, among those who know of it, who would prefer the hospital. If you were the CEO of hospital A, you have reason to rejoice. But if you are with hospitals G or H, alarm bells should be sounding. You may have substantial problems with consumers, problems that forecast a decline in the hospital's census.

If a hospital asked for your financial help, what are the chances that you would contribute?
Definitely would contribute 14%
Maybe 48%
Definitely would not
   contribute 38%

Have you ever contributed money to a hospital?
Yes 15%
No...................... 85%

The responses to the foregoing questions show that most people are aware of several hospitals in the market area. Nearly everyone has selected the hospital he expects to use in advance. Thus, consumer preferences are highly developed. The follow-up question indicates a far wider base of support for the hospitals' fund-raising efforts than might be thought likely.

The data may also reflect a more loyal following for individual hospitals than HSAs are aware of. The number of respondents who said they would consider a contribution if asked for help far exceeded the number of persons who said they had ever contributed to a hospital.

Measuring the Attitudes of Doctors and Nurses

At one time or another, many hospitals find themselves making big decisions about their medical staffs with too little information. Even if data were readily available, however, each hospital should do its own study because hospital staffs differ so widely from one another.

This chapter presents samples of questions that hospitals have used in their quest for better information about their medical and nursing staffs and that illustrate the kind of findings you might be interested in knowing for your own hospital. The findings that follow are from a study done for a Midwest area hospital in 1978.

Listed below are attributes that hospitals may or may not have. How do you rate the importance or the desirability of each of these in hospitals with which you like to be affiliated?

Mean Rating (High = 9; Low = 1)

Attribute	Staff Members	Prospects
Private office	7.50	7.46
Adjacent or nearby location	7.30	6.88
Close friendships	6.35	6.60
Friendly, congenial atmosphere	5.31	5.84
Medical school affiliation	1.84	1.89
Outpatient services	7.62	7.36
Low cost to patients	6.65	5.46
Single-room wing	3.74	3.79
Public admissions policy of nondiscrimination	6.89	6.07
Prestigious public image	3.22	3.00

The research found big differences in which aspects of the hospital doctors valued. This enabled the hospital to concentrate on those services that were important to doctors. By also surveying doctors whom the hospital was trying to attract to its medical staff, the survey was able to relate directly to physicians' interests. Note the greatest importance attached to the attributes of outpatient services and office space by both medical staff members and by prospects.

Hospitals also worry and make important decisions about their nursing staffs. The same hospital management that decided it needed to know more about its medical staff also decided to find out more about its nurses. Nursing staffs, like medical staffs, vary considerably in their attitudes from hospital to hospital; so do the talent pools from which the nursing staff is drawn. The data that follow are from a research study conducted in 1979.

If you decided to work here, how much would you expect to earn an hour? How would you rate your chances of taking a job if it paid 50 cents an hour more than that offered by other nearby hospitals?

Current Setting of Working Nurses	Expected Wage per Hour	Percent Influenced by 50 Cents/Hr. Differential
Hospital	$9.04	14%
Nursing Home	$9.14	17%
Doctor's office	$8.97	17%
Nurse not working	$8.87	16%

The study of nurses living in the area served by this hospital found that salary expectations were generally quite similar, regardless of where a nurse worked or whether she was employed. The study also found that for most nurses a pay scale 50 cents above the norm did little to attract them. This helped the hospital to concentrate on other areas besides pay in its recruiting program and in its efforts to retain nurses already working at the facility.

Observations about Consumer Research

It is not likely that you will either want to dig or should dig deeply into the technicalities of the consumer research process, because that is the domain of the professional researcher. It may help, however, if you understand a few basic tools of research and a little of the researcher's vocabulary.

Sample Size. The measurement of public opinion requires talking to samples of the population, not talking to the whole population that interest you. How big should the sample be? Use the smallest sample size that will give you reliable data. On a relatively small sample, a useful rule of thumb is to not expand the sample size if the results are on the order of 75:25. For example:

- If you ask 100 persons a question in a properly selected sample, and the answers are 75 "for" and 25 "opposed," it is likely that even if you expanded the size of your sample to 1,000 respondents, the results would still be in the range of 70:30 to 80:20.
- If you ask 100 persons a question and the answers are 52 "for" and 48 "opposed," you may need to ask 10,000 people in order to be confident that you have an accurate estimate. Often, you can get by with small samples—and that keeps the cost down.

Common Sense. Use your consumer research dollars carefully. Spend big on important issues, spend small on lesser issues.

Focus Groups. This is a useful research technique to help plan studies that you may hear about if your hospital becomes involved in consumer research. A trained discussion leader spends two or three hours with 8 or 10 selected persons talking about subjects of interest to your hospital. The discussion leader should not be identified with your hospital.

Focus groups provide a way to find out what issues to raise, how to raise them, and what language consumers use. The technique is also a way to develop ideas and answers to problems. For instance, if the marketing director were contemplating a new system of directional signs in the hospital, it would be instructive for the hospital management to listen to a focus group to learn the words that consumers use to describe different parts of the hospital. Managers of consumer-oriented businesses frequently attend focus groups to open their eyes and minds to "real" consumers and how they talk about the company's products. It is a way to keep close to what people have on their minds as opposed to what management *thinks* they have on their minds.

Another technique is to make a videotape of the focus group, and then edit the tape to 30 minutes (screening out the garbage) and play it to wider audiences. For instance, the videotape of a group talking about the behavior of physicians in the hospital, the business office, or the parking conditions could be the basis for discussion and instruction in your hospital.

Now here is a warning about focus groups: the flip side is that the information cannot be used as data. The group is too small, it is always biased, and it has been conditioned by the leader and other members. Focus groups have validity as a preliminary step. They should never be substituted for quantifiable research.

Proprietary Information. Much consumer research measures public opinion on sensitive issues. Even though the research is done to improve the decisions you make on the public's behalf, that does not mean you should go public with all the information you gather. You will want to keep some of it, probably most of it, private.

Pooling Research Dollars with Other Hospitals. Occasionally there will be research projects of common interest among a group of hospitals. This suggests joint research and lowered cost to each hospital. The trouble with these projects is that they demand much time to organize. Getting the managements, the boards of trustees, and the medical staffs of six hospitals to agree on a research project usually turns out to be just about impossible. However, if it can be put together, some real dollars can be saved.

Wrapping It Up. In summary, you should recognize that consumer research

- Costs money, and must be budgeted
- Needs careful planning
- Is an area of expertise in which you should not play amateur-hour games

It is the hospital's obligation to measure public opinion before important decisions are made and, after the fact, to measure the hospital's performance so that improvements can be made.

The Key Question about Research

The key question the management and the board of each hospital must ask itself now is this: how long can our hospital continue without the kind of data illustrated in the previous chapters? The data are real. The hospitals that commissioned the studies are already well into the "marketing age," using market research to improve their decision-making capabilities.

Some of the research was commissioned by a hospital board member, some by a CEO, some by a hospital director of planning. The spread of subjects that were researched and are described is quite wide: information of use to the public policy maker, insights for the marketing director, data for a hospital with medical staff recruiting problems, data for nurse recruitment. And almost all of the data are useful to the planning director.

Marketing research is useful to the hospital. It will help the hospital make better decisions. From the perspective of our whole society, that is good news because consumers' interests will be better served. Some hospitals are already breaking the trail. It seems likely that no hospital can ignore powerful tools like these and remain competitive for long.

Market Positioning and Impression Statements

Market Positioning Expresses the Hospital's Mission

In the annual marketing plan outlined earlier, the importance of the market positioning, or impression statements, was discussed. The market positioning is drawn from the mission statement and describes what your hospital stands for.

What *does* your hospital stand for? Until you can answer that with precision, the hospital's marketing program is in trouble. Until all the individual doctors, nurses, department heads, and trustees can answer it with a single voice, you have confusion and are giving the public mixed signals.

What do you stand for? How you choose to answer that question is just about the whole ball game. Among marketing people, it is called *positioning*. Positioning is best explained by demonstration. Some examples of positionings:

- "We are the only hospital within 100 miles of where you are standing."
- "We specialize in the treatment of eye diseases. Only eyes, nothing but eyes, and we are the best on the Eastern seaboard."
- "Our hospital is attached to a huge medical school, and its primary mission is the training of physicians."
- "We are a nursing home dedicated to the care of senile, confused patients."
- "We are an extended care hospital whose role is to care for terminally ill cancer patients."

Each of these facilities has a clear positioning. A single sentence describes what it is and what it stands for. Every doctor, every employee, and every patient can understand the facility's role in the community. Communication on every front can be effective. Marketing these institutions is, or should be, simple because there is a clear positioning that grows directly from each institution's decision about what it chooses to be.

Here is another positioning: "Loving Arms is a medium-sized community hospital that offers much the same services as the other hospitals around here." Think about this statement for a moment. Unfortunately, it is how many of the trustees, CEOs, and doctors view their hospitals, and *that* is a problem. Most hospitals fall into the middle range in size, and most are not easily distinguishable from competitive hospitals. The staffs and trustees do not understand the differences, so of course patients cannot distinguish them meaningfully either. This is where marketing techniques will help the most, and it is where the public can be helped the most.

Hospitals that appear to be undifferentiated from all the alternatives are probably most susceptible to "bed cutting."

If you do not develop and explain a distinctive positioning for your hospital, then you are just part of a pool of beds. The public has an interest in this, of course, if it is about to lose a facility it values. It also has a vital interest in knowing just what the hospital does stand for. So your hospital has the obligation to understand its own positioning and to communicate it effectively.

The public has no problem understanding the hospital whose positioning is "We are the only hospital within 100 miles." In a case of need, it is clear that this is the place to go. But the positioning isn't all that clear at most hospitals. From now on, we'll address the problem of these undifferentiated hospitals.

The Hospital's Positioning: You Do Not Invent It, You Discover It

The positioning of your hospital must be real, not imagined; you are going to market real services, real skills, and real equipment and facilities. The positioning you adopt must be discovered in the realities of the hospital itself, not invented. Newcomers to this process often stall at this point, toss in the towel, and are inclined to say, "We are all pretty much alike," a statement that almost always turns out to be untrue.

Hospitals are *not* created equal. They are quite different from one another, and your job is to discover how your hospital can be distinguished from others in your community. Here is how you go about finding the differences that are important in the proper positioning of your hospital. As a starter, ask yourself these questions:

- *What is the size (in beds) of our hospital compared with the size of consumers' alternative choices?*
  - —This might be the information that leads to the positioning of "the biggest hospital with the broadest range of services."
  - —Or, it may lead to the positioning that the hospital is "small but with a high level of personal nursing service."
- *What medical facilities might separate us from the alternative hospitals?*
  - —Are our emergency facilities different? Bigger, smaller, newer, better?
  - —Do we have a key group of specialists at our hospital?
  - —Do we treat a particular disease more often than the other hospitals?
  - —Do we have more single-bed rooms?
  - —Is nursing care demonstrably different?
  - —Are we strong as a rehabilitation hospital?
  - —Do we have the biggest psychiatric unit in the city?
  - —Is our substance abuse treatment program more effective, bigger, or longer established?
  - —Does our program of education distinguish us?
  - —Do we have a famous physician on the staff?

What you are looking for in the answers to these questions are the medically based areas of strengths, the things that help distinguish your hospital from your competitors.

- *How does our location make us different from other hospitals?*
  - —Are we close to a freeway exit?
  - —Are we in a downtown location or at the hub of the transportation system?
  - —Are we next to a big regional shopping center?
  - —Are we in a densely populated area?
  - —Do we have plenty of easily accessible parking?
  - —Are we next to the city's best-known landmark?
  - —Are we in a small-town setting?

If any of these descriptions apply to your hospital, you should let your potential customers know how your hospital is different from others in the area.

- *How does the management of our hospital make us different?*
  - —Have we pioneered new systems?
  - —Is our business office the most efficient, most professional, least bureaucratic, most sensible, or most friendly in town?
  - —Have we got the lowest room rates?
  - —Do we lead in the effort to slow the rise in hospital costs?
  - —Do we have individuals in management who are unusually active in a hospital association or who are recognized regionally or nationally for their work in a hospital association?
  - —Have any of our staff members had a paper published in a professional journal or do they consult with other hospitals?

Strengths in management, particularly strengths that contribute to either more effective service to patients or cost control, have increasing relevance in today's economic environment. So a reputation for effective management and sensible and friendly customer relations in the business office may be strengths to build on.

- *How does our long-range plan make us different?*
  - —Are we going to move the hospital?
  - —Are we going to merge it?
  - —Are we going to expand an area of service or improve it?
  - —Are we converting from one level of care to another?
  - —Are we (or is the health systems agency in the area) planning to designate our hospital as a regional center for pediatrics or emergency service, or as a burn center?

Your hospital's positioning should be consonant with the long-range plan, and if big changes are in store, they must be reflected by the positioning.

- *How does the religious heritage of your hospital affect consumers' choices?* Some research indicates:
  —Catholic hospitals are thought to be more caring.
  —Jewish hospitals are thought to have more specialists on the staff.
  —Nonsectarian hospitals are likely to charge you more.

What is there about the religious heritage of your hospital that belongs in the positioning? Although it seems to be popular today to deny the religious heritage of the hospital, research shows that the religious background of the hospital does indeed influence consumers' choice of hospital.

This list of starter questions is designed to help you ferret out the strengths of your hospital and discover its market positioning. Knowing your strengths is important to you. It is also important to consumers who make decisions about your hospital. They are entitled to know; you are obligated to communicate.

Note that you have not been asked to be creative, innovative, or fanciful. You don't invent your positioning; you discover it by uncovering all of the facts about your hospital. You have this aspect of your marketing effort under control if, when someone asks you what your hospital is all about, you can respond unhesitatingly and clearly in three sentences—and the same question, when put to three other representatives of the hospital, produces the same response.

Alternative Positionings

The market positioning you identify for your hospital must be true, brief, and believable. In addition, if the positioning is to be effective, it should be interesting or have a small edge of surprise that makes it memorable.

Here is the cocktail party test for market positioning. If someone asks, "What do you do?," you can answer, "I am a hospital administrator." That's true, brief, and believable. You could also answer, "I am the chief executive officer of Loving Arms Hospital." You have now added importance to the position and made your description more specific. Finally, you could answer, "I am the chief executive officer of Loving Arms Hospital and the guy responsible for raising the rates last month!" At that point, you have probably selected a position that will get you some attention. That's what "edge of surprise" means. You are seeking not only a market positioning that describes the hospital, but also ways to state the hospital's positioning that attract interest and attention.

Now take a look at some of the choices you have. For the same 300-bed hospital each of these positionings could be written.

Positioning 1: We're the hospital that's easy to reach in times of emergency or to visit someone at. Once you get there you can find a parking place, and it is easy to get around. Everything is so convenient.

This is the convenience positioning. In a crowded city with many hospitals, it might be an important positioning you could adopt.

Positioning 2: Our strength is the teaching medical staff. We have many specialists, most of them engaged in teaching residents and interns. That's good for patients, because it means that the most up-to-date methods and techniques are used.

This is the medical specialist positioning. It can be refined much further, of course, to specialists in cancer or heart surgery, and so on. This positioning may be useful in differentiating the hospital as the right place to go for the treatment of serious illness.

Positioning 3: We are a Catholic hospital where Christian care by the nursing staff, in support of the physicians, has been the practice for 75 years.
This is the Christian care position.

Each of these statements describes the same hospital. The question is, which describes the hospital most accurately and most advantageously? Many hospital personnel will answer, "Let's use all three." In fact, you might be able to do so. The trouble is that the more content you pack into the description of the market positioning, the more difficult communication becomes. And communication is what marketing is all about. Usually, you have to choose and trade off some content in favor of communication.

Now, what about those three alternatives? Which is best? The answer is, it depends. It depends on how many competitors your hospital faces and what their positionings are. It depends on how consumers view what is important to them and on what is missing in the array of choices they have.

The way to find out the power of an array of positionings is to "try it out on the dog." You assess the relative value of each positioning by using marketing research techniques. You get the answer by asking the persons you want to communicate with. You do *not* ask your associates at the hospital or your friends. They all think as you do.

In reprise, the market positioning is:

- A summary statement of what the hospital wants communicated
- The distilled essence of what the hospital is, very much like the mission statement in the hospital's long-range plan
- The platform on which all communication will be built—the public statements made by officials of the hospital, the annual report, all patient communication, all graphics, advertising, and so on.

When you have correctly identified your market positioning and have done the job well, you have accomplished much. Everything else will flow from this essential step.

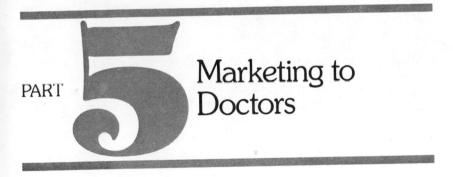

PART **5** Marketing to Doctors

Stereotypes
and Communication

Physicians are much like everyone else. They generally behave quite predictably: they react positively to some stimuli, negatively to others. Far from being curmudgeonish, unpredictable, hard to get at, or difficult to communicate with (the stereotype built around them), they are, or can be, among the easiest groups to deal with. Physicians usually pick up all the cues and signals, quickly comprehending the subtleties and inconsistencies of any communication that deals with their profession.

Many hospital administrators find it difficult to get doctors to respond positively to their hospital's plans, and many hospital trustees and administrators list this as the number one ongoing, unsolved problem their hospitals face. It is in such hospitals that the administrator's relationship with the medical staff could be dramatically improved if the administrator could capture and use some very ordinary marketing skills.

Many CEOs and trustees are cynical about doctors' motivations and, interestingly, so are a lot of doctors. Many stereotypes are in wide use; among them are the following:

- The trouble with doctors is that all they think of is money.
- The trouble with doctors is that they don't know anything about management and meeting a payroll. (There are a considerable number of doctors who are managing a bigger payroll and a higher overhead structure than many trustees.)
- The trouble with doctors is that all they do is take from the hospital and never put anything back. (Many doctors put in much time in staff and committee meetings at their hospitals, and the medical staff turns out to be generous when fund drives are on.)

These stereotypes are resented by physicians, and with reason. Like most stereotypes, they often are unfair, inaccurate, and break down fast under examination. It is these stereotypes that get in the way of communication, which is essential to marketing. Good communication with physicians, or effective marketing, begins with an under-standing, and there is no great science in understanding what makes physicians tick—just horse sense and some elementary skills.

Straight Talk about Doctors

Many hospital trustees and management people regard marketing to doctors as a hazardous occupation that probably should be rewarded with combat pay. Only a fearless survivor of many encounters with physicians would dare to offer the following observations on physicians:

- Physicians, just like everyone else, want your respect. They want to feel that you are dealing with them as individuals of importance and not as a part of a stereotype that you have in your head. Examine your own attitudes when you feel hostility and surliness coming at you from physicians.
- Patient care is the "hot button." The overwhelming majority of physicians are concerned about patients and the care they get. This concern is genuine and deep. It is the single biggest hot button you can push. They usually respond well to proposals that result in better patient care, provided they understand them.
- Understand that as a group, physicians are just as diverse and perverse as your board of trustees. They have different reading tastes, different interests in sports, different interests in art, different musical tastes, different hobbies, and drive different brands of cars. Don't underestimate how many different perceptions or how many different results can be triggered by a single hospital communication.
- Physicians, like the rest of us, would rather be a little rich than a little poor. Things that affect the wallet are highly sensitive. Unlike the rest of us, however, many have trouble admitting that out loud to lay people. The result is that only rarely will they admit to voting no on a proposal because it would cut into their income. Usually, the reason given is that they are opposed for patient care reasons (a socially acceptable reason), or they just feel curmudgeonish that day.
- Physicians generally come equipped with big egos, developed by the intense survival course they went through on the way to

becoming a doctor. The course was tough, and they know it. They want to think that you know it, too.

- Most physicians do not like change. Almost nobody accepts change gracefully, physicians probably least of all. Deal with this firmly, but with exquisite care. In a changing structure of social values, physicians in private practice may well be the last to change. They are among the last of the free enterprisers, the biggest group of practicing, card-carrying capitalists in the country, and most still believe in the ethic of hard work.

There was a reason for running through that list. The observations can be distilled into a few, but important points to keep in mind when marketing to physicians. When you run into problems with the medical staff, consider that it might be your fault. Treat the physicians with respect in your marketing efforts, and treat them with candor and honesty in your communications.

Get the hospital's act together so that everyone is working together. Physicians will be the first to note conflicting signals. Every communication to physicians should be examined through the eyes of the physician intensely interested in the quality of care his or her patients get. Don't threaten the physician's standard of living with careless moves that reduce his or her income.

Physicians are an important audience for a hospital's marketing effort.

Researching Physician Attitudes

Most hospitals correctly identify a need to market to doctors. Among the most common problems marketing is called upon to help solve are:

- Recruiting physicians to the medical staff
- Persuading physicians on the staff who practice at other hospitals to send more patients to your hospital
- Convincing physicians that they should join trustees and management in a cause or an endeavor (like a building-fund campaign or politicking with a local agency)

There are several reasons why these marketing efforts directed to physicians often prove fruitless. The most common one is that the marketing program began with answers and not with questions. Before running ads in medical society journals and newsletters seeking to recruit doctors, you should be surveying the medical staff to find out why you are having problems in the first place.

One Eastern hospital spent 18 months and a large sum of money recruiting internists, but with no results. At that time, it was discovered that the single principal reason the hospital could not attract internists was the chief of internal medicine himself. The recruiting effort was successful in attracting interest, but no one signed up. The reason: the chief wanted the referrals himself and was methodically turning the candidates off as each inquired about joining the staff. A small survey of the medical staff uncovered that fact after considerable effort had been wasted.

Before marketing anything of consequence to doctors, it is a good idea to find out what the obstacles are. Sometimes you can learn what they are by talking to individual staff members over coffee or lunch. However, if the issue is a big one, or if it is sensitive, you will want to use professional survey research, because the doctors who are the source of the information you need must feel free to give honest answers without the fear of recriminations. Only professional research can provide the anonymity that candid expression may require.

For example, your question to a doctor who practices at another hospital might be "Why are your admissions declining at our hospital?" Asked face-to-face, the response is likely to be risk-free:

- "I am changing the emphasis of my practice."
- "This hospital has always been my first choice, but I am taking it a little easier now."

Or the question may provide an opening for ax grinding and produce responses such as these:

- "I told you three years ago we need a better-equipped doctors' lounge."
- "The other hospital provides me with secretarial services."

The professional researcher can protect the doctors' identities so that they are able to answer with candor and confidence and might respond this way:

- "Admissions to this hospital are being reduced because I have more confidence in the nursing staff at Hospital B."
- "I disagree with the policies of this hospital's board and am increasing my involvement at Hospital B."
- "I do not have confidence in the chief of my department."
- "The other hospital is able to provide coverage for my patients on weekends and nights."

In large hospitals, the professional researcher will be able to survey more physicians on the staff than the administration would have time for. That is another reason why he should be able to provide more accurate measurements of the medical staff's attitudes. When the stakes are big, marketing to doctors begins with research and with questions, not with answers.

Debunking the Myth
That Only Doctors
Influence Hospital Choice

Many hospital trustees have been told (frequently in commanding tones of voice) by physicians, administrators, other trustees, and even marketing academics that "everyone knows that physicians, not patients, select the hospital." The extension of this belief is the conclusion that "you market the hospital to doctors, not to patients." But studies of the process by which consumers select a hospital lend neither credence nor comfort to the conventional wisdom of the industry, which, in effect, says you cannot control the destiny of your hospital except through the medical staff.

The studies tracked the decision-making process of 198 patients in the Twin Cities, another 400 patients in Chicago, and 432 patients selected on a national basis.* Here is what those consumers said about how they selected a hospital:

- 50 to 67 percent (depending on which study) say, sure enough, that the doctor picked the hospital.
- 30 to 45 percent say that they themselves selected the hospital. They did it by selecting the hospital first and getting the physician as a result, or selecting the physician because they knew that he was on the staff of a hospital they preferred.
- 13 to 18 percent said they would change doctors if he left the staff of "their" hospital.

The significance of the data is important. It means that (1) although the doctors are very important, the board of trustees and the administration are *not* totally dependent on the medical staff for the hospital's business; (2) consumers are exercising choice far more than was believed by almost all "experts"; and (3) marketing to a broad public, as opposed to the simpler concept of "marketing to doctors," has great relevance to hospitals in the '80s.

The knowledge that consumers are important in the process of

---

*Studies conducted in 1977-1980 by Leo J. Shapiro and Associates, Inc., Chicago.

selecting a hospital is what makes marketing an important subject to hospitals at this time. Because consumers think they have a vote, it is up to you to express what you stand for. That's what marketing is all about.

In addition, there is evidence that suggests a growing awareness among consumers that they can influence the cost and quality of health care by the selections they make among doctors, hospitals, and other health care providers. Look at the growth in a two-year period in the number of people who say that their choice of health care provider does make a difference in costs, as shown in the following questions from studies conducted in 1975 and 1977.

Speaking about the costs of medical care, does the health provider that you choose make any difference in the cost of your medical care?

	Percent Who Say Yes		
	May '75	May '77	Net Difference
Doctor that you choose affects the cost of your medical care	28%	31%	+3%
Dentist that you choose affects the cost of your dental care	30%	29%	(−1%)
Hospital that you go to affects the cost of your hospital care	20%	25%	+5%
Medical and x-ray lab that you go to or that your doctor chooses affects the cost of your medical tests	15%	23%	+8%
Insurance company that you buy from affects the cost of health insurance protection	30%	36%	+6%
Drugstore that you go to affects the cost of prescriptions	49%	45%	(−4%)

The data suggest that consumers are tending to be more aware and more sensitive to health care costs and the possibilities for influencing their own expenditures on them. The data could also be interpreted to mean that consumers are feeling steadily less helpless or less dependent on decisions made by others.

The response to another question from the same studies shows a growing conviction among consumers that the choice of provider can make a lot of difference in the *quality* of the care received.

Costs aside, does the health provider that you choose make any difference in the quality of your medical care?

	Percent Who Say Yes		
	May '75	May '77	Net Difference
Doctor that you choose affects the quality of your medical care	52%	63%	+11%
Dentist that you choose affects the quality of your dental care	49%	58%	+ 9%
Hospital that you go to affects the quality of your hospital care	38%	54%	+16%
Medical and x-ray lab that you go to or your doctor chooses affects the quality of your medical care	30%	42%	+12%
Insurance company you buy from affects the quality of health insurance protection	37%	48%	+11%
Drugstore that you go to affects the quality of prescriptions	33%	43%	+10%

So much for the belief that hospitals need only to market to doctors! Consumers are demonstrating through these data an increased involvement in the medical decision-making process.

The balanced view you should carry forward from this chapter is that doctors are an important audience to the hospital and cannot be ignored. Yet consumers are also important—and undoubtedly getting steadily more important. Long ignored, they must now be front and center in your marketing activities; often they will be the key. And there are also legislators, board members of the various agencies of government, and the bureaucrats who also must be influenced.

PART **6** Public Relations

Public Relations: Separating the Fantasy from the Fact

The role of public relations is to help the hospital get its story across to its various publics, and it is one of the key tools in the marketing arsenal. The hospital cannot afford second-rate performance in this activity. Unfortunately, many CEOs, board members, and doctors operate in a fantasy land concerning public relations activities, so it may be useful to describe some basic facts about PR, its advantages and disadvantages.

A great advantage is that the hospital does not pay for space in the newspaper or the exposure it gets on radio or television. The space or time is free. (Of course, the cost of running the PR department is *not* free.)

Another big advantage of effective PR is that a story about your hospital under the banner of the newspaper or TV news will be more widely believed than when it appears on your own letterhead. When the hospital's message appears in the news column, it takes on some of the credibility of that medium.

But a hospital cannot control *exactly* how the message will come out, even in really first-rate, professionally run media. All you can do is suggest; you cannot control the message with precision. That's the big disadvantage of PR—and a major advantage of advertising.

The message: the PR activity can deliver a lot of value, but it should be understood as an instrument with limitations.

Problems Begin with Trustees and CEOs

It is a rare hospital whose public relations function is really performing to potential. Usually, there are two problems. The first is a simple lack of knowledge in hospitals about how journalists and the media work. And that leads to considerable naivete about what to expect of the PR function. The second problem is the lack of a marketing plan, which means that the PR department is usually operating with considerably less than clear direction. The frequent result is that the PR efforts are sporadic and usually concentrate on emergency situations only, rather than on clearly established objectives.

Another problem is that hospital management and boards of trustees simply have not provided the kind of leadership or the kind of climate that would allow the PR function to perform effectively. The problem can be illustrated with some direct quotations gleaned from hospital CEOs over the past few years. The comments are on the left, and some observations about them are on the right.

Quotations from Hospital Management	Observations
Newspapers are the most important news medium.	Newspapers are indeed important, but most consumers get their news from television and radio.
Reporters and the news media do not use the handouts we provide, which proves that they are biased.	If anything, this proves lack of bias. You wouldn't want to read or see news that is composed mostly of partisan public relations releases. A news medium that accepts your release in toto is probably doing the same with everything else it receives.
The other hospitals get much better press coverage than we do.	Possibly they have built better relationships with the media. Perhaps they answered the calls of

	reporters faster. They may have been more open, more honest, or have said more newsworthy things.
I urged them to kill a story because it was untrue and would damage the hospital.	This is a classic example of PR ineptitude. Trying to kill a story almost guarantees that the reporter will pursue it harder, dig deeper, and call the opposition for further comment.
I pointed out a great story about our new laundry, and they wouldn't print it.	Maybe the story was not framed in a way that made it news. Maybe it was a dull story in the first place. Maybe your story landed on the reporter's desk in the middle of a day when hard news was breaking.
The TV interview lasted for an hour, and only a 30-second quote, which was totally out of context, was used.	This frequently heard comment exhibits real naivete about the construction of broadcast news programming. Only the president of the United States gets quoted more than that. The secret is to learn how to give memorable 30-second replies instead of sermons.
They never call us to get our side of a story.	Maybe this is because you haven't answered their calls before, because they can never get through to you, or because you are always in meetings. Perhaps they simply don't know that you exist. Possibly you need to visit the reporters in your town so that they know you by sight and know that you are a good guy.

Each of these quotations indicates a problem concerning knowledge of PR activities.

The public relations function is destined to get even more important in the age of marketing. To make its full contribution, however, it will need to be managed by CEOs whose knowledge of PR is substantially greater than that generally seen in the hospital today. Also needed is an appropriately staffed department; in some cases this will mean a higher grade of personnel will be needed. Finally, PR departments will need to operate within a framework of a full marketing plan.

The next chapters present a primer for CEOs; guidelines on staffing, especially the relationship of the PR director to the marketing director; and the objectives of a PR program. Because of their importance, the PR "disaster plan" and the stress interview are also discussed in this part of the book.

A Primer for CEOs

To the consternation of their competitors, some hospitals consistently get favorable treatment in the press. These hospitals have effective public relations. Effective PR is neither mysterious nor very difficult. Because PR is important to the total marketing effort, this brief primer will be useful to hospital CEOs:

1. The management team needs to be working within a marketing strategy. It also must have the hospital's mission statement and market positioning firmly in mind. If the hospital has a clear-cut positioning, the hospital spokesman or representative will always be able to get the message into the answer, no matter what the reporter asks.
2. The CEO must be willing to work at the job, taking guidance from his PR professionals, meeting reporters, answering their calls and questions, and seeking them out if they do not call. It takes time and effort, but most of all, it takes desire.
3. The representative must start with respect for and an understanding of the journalist's needs. The reporter's objective is a news story that the editor will judge to be worth using. Generally, that means a story that *many* consumers will find interesting. The hospital representative should respect the reporter's time and the fact that the reporter is working on deadlines a few minutes or a few hours away. This is why reporters sometimes appear pushy.
4. If the hospital wants to comment on a story, calls from reporters should be answered immediately. Failure to respond is the same as giving up the chance to influence what is going to be said about your hospital. Failure to respond also allows reporters to say, "Officials at Loving Arms Hospital could not be reached for comment."
5. The hospital representative must not say, "No comment." There are very few occasions when a hospital can say, "No comment" and not lose. "No comment" is viewed as the language of persons who have something to hide, even if that is not true.

6. The hospital representative must be honest, open, and candid; it shows. He or she should not be afraid to say, "We were wrong." The representative should not even be afraid to say, "We try hard, but as in all human enterprises, mistakes are made occasionally. This one was a real dilly." Reporters and readers alike will empathize with the representative's embarrassment. Reporters will sense a coverup or a lack of candor 10 times out of 10.
7. Never bluff when you don't have the facts. It is always acceptable to say, "I don't know the answer to that, but I'll check." When you do this, be sure to ask what the reporter's deadline is, and then follow up.
8. Nothing is ever off the record when talking to a reporter. Don't say anything you do not want to see printed or broadcast.

Of course, what this short PR primer adds up to is really just good human relations. Unfortunately, a perfectly nice person sometimes turns into someone not so nice when a reporter comes to ask questions.

There are reasons for a negative reaction. Sometimes the CEO has been burned and is scared. Sometimes he does not respect the reporter's job and shows it. Sometimes the CEO has not been adequately briefed about how to deal with the press, so he falls apart in crises (which means that something very newsworthy is happening). Last, the CEO may have no plan and no program of positive action and therefore is always on the defensive, always on the run; it shows.

From PR to Marketing: Making the Transition

The public relations department in most hospitals currently carries the main burden for marketing. Public relations is a subset of marketing, but the two activities are not the same. Marketing is not just a new name for what the PR director has been doing for the hospital. Many hospitals already have a PR practitioner on staff. What does he or she need to make the transition to marketing?

Some hospital PR directors already have the skills to direct a hospital's marketing efforts, but many do not. If a hospital contemplates promoting its PR practitioner to the job of marketing director, it should assess the PR practitioner's business skills, background in consumer research, knowledge of advertising, and familiarity with graphics and design.

Many public relations persons do not get much exposure to hospital finance and management because their activities are regarded as special and off the beaten track by hospital management. The result is that ordinary business skills are sometimes lacking. Adequate business skills are necessary to carry out a marketing program.

Many persons in hospital management, including PR practitioners, do not have a background in consumer research. Numerous courses and seminars exist to help correct this deficiency, however. If the PR person is to successfully make the transition to marketing, he or she must pick up some rudimentary skills in this area.

Advertising is another subject in which public relations practitioners generally have only slight expertise. However, the transition to marketing director will require that they be conversant in several areas: how to select the right medium, how to develop the advertising message, how to get the message together mechanically, and so on. These skills can be learned, but the need to learn them must be recognized and addressed. Creating good advertising requires new skills.

Design and graphics is a subject about which most persons know far less than they think. Buying graphics and design is one of the shakiest areas of marketing for two reasons: many buyers are amateurs, and many sellers are giving you their own ego needs. Getting graphics that work to support your marketing strategy is not as easy as saying, "I know what I like." It is a talent that the PR practitioner will need in the marketing job.

Skills in these four areas are most likely to be the ones that a public relations practitioner needs to improve or polish in order to succeed as a hospital's principal marketing mover. But there are other needs as well, such as temperament and ego.

A successful marketing person is results-oriented; he or she is competitive and plays to win. This person also needs to be tough enough and confident enough to challenge the CEO, the doctors, and the board of trustees—few of whom have highly developed marketing skills and many of whom may react negatively to direction from marketing persons. The public relations person who is to make the transition to marketing director must also be disciplined enough to reject "gofer" work that others in the hospital may try to push on him or her; otherwise, there will be neither time nor stature to achieve marketing success.

The person who handles marketing for your hospital must constantly examine the hospital's actions from the point of view of an "inside-consumer," someone who can anticipate the reactions of consumers and do something to prevent mistakes. That takes a special person who will read every memo, listen to every statement, observe every action, and (constantly siding with consumers) raise hell *before* the public hears about it. That is a special talent.

Finally, the marketing person should be a capable representative of the hospital and be able to teach others to be effective in that role. All of these qualities go into the marketing director's job description. Until the PR person can meet them, he or she is not qualified.

Objectives for the PR Director

Building effective public relations is one of those jobs that requires steady hard work. It isn't a problem that you solve once and then forget. Good PR comes when the hospital management values it enough to put it high on the list of hospital priorities, provides a marketing plan so that clear direction is present for the activity, ensures an adequate budget so that the objectives set out in the marketing plan can be met, and makes sure someone who knows the ropes is working to achieve the objectives.

Most of the PR effort must be delegated to the PR staff. For the benefit of those who have no background in this activity, here are the nine basic objectives of an effective program, objectives that the CEO and the PR director should be working together to achieve:

1. *Develop and periodically update a press kit of background materials about the hospital for use with the media.* At a minimum, the press kit should include the following:

   - Names of those who are designated by the hospital to meet and deal with the press
   - The hospital's mission statement
   - The annual report
   - A list of the trustees
   - A list of the management of the hospital
   - A list of the physicians who practice at the hospital
   - A chronology of significant events in the hospital's history, usually about two or three pages in length
   - A fact sheet listing the facility's location, number of beds, medical specialties, and principal areas of strength
   - A generalized press release about the hospital
   - Glossy photos of the CEO, the board president, and the president of the medical staff

2. *Develop and keep current a list of all the news media of importance to the hospital.* The hospital's PR department should have accurate,

current names of the reporters who cover hospital news. It should also know the names of those consumer advocates who cover consumer news. The list must be kept current; reporters' assignments are frequently changed.

3. *Designate who is the authorized spokesman for the hospital.* The hospital must make sure that reporters have been informed, and it must make certain that internal procedures are in place so that everyone around the hospital knows how to refer press inquiries to the proper spokesman. The hospital's representatives must, of course, be listed in the order of the hospital's preference, so that everyone knows which person to get to. If this is not done, a diligent reporter will always get to someone, and that will almost always turn out to be the wrong one from the hospital's standpoint.

4. *The PR person should make periodic visits to each reporter who handles hospital news in the hospital's area.* Remember to include broadcast media. Meetings can be arranged at a breakfast or a lunch, although this isn't essential. The purposes of these visits are modest and include the following:

   - The hospital needs to get to know the reporters.
   - The hospital wants to ensure that the press kit is in each medium's background files so that when the heat is on, each has a good data base from which to work. It is important that neither the medium nor the hospital is scrambling in the middle of a news crisis.
   - The PR person wants to set a date for the reporter to come and see the hospital firsthand, tour the facilities, and get to know the place and the personnel.

5. *Create and place positive news stories.* This is a big reason for an active PR operation, and it includes the creation of the story, taking pictures, and getting the story to the media. The hospital will do better, however, when the PR person selects a specific reporter who is likely to be interested and then arranges an interview with the proper spokesman at the hospital. Another way to achieve this objective is to arrange for one of the hospital's officers to make a speech and report the story "as delivered to _____."

6. *Learn to be opportunistic.* The organization that believes public relations is valuable always finds many opportunities to make news. If your hospital works at it, it is not hard to be steadily in the news.

7. *Help the hospital's CEO become the industry spokesman in your town.* Local reporters need local authorities to quote. When some big shot in Washington makes a statement, the reporter often wants

to localize the story. The hospital CEO who is known to local reporters, and who has proven to be an ally by always responding to calls, is halfway home to having the hospital's name in the paper or being mentioned on the evening news.

8. *Learn to say things in a newsworthy way.* This is how you achieve industry representative status. Let us assume that Senator Kennedy has just made a statement in Washington, and a reporter calls two local hospitals and talks to their CEOs. One of the CEOs responds by saying, "Senator Kennedy is entitled to his views, of course, but there is a contrary view espoused by the House of Delegates of the State Hospital Association, which on six separate occasions noted these flaws in that position." The other CEO responds by saying, "Senator Kennedy is an economics illiterate." Both CEOs have said the same thing, but only one will be quoted. Only one will be called back. Only one will become the industry representative.

9. *Develop a PR disaster plan.* The components of such a plan are described in the next chapter.

What we have described here are the rudiments of a PR program that will work. Good PR, like most jobs, is about 1 percent PR genius, 48 percent creating and adhering to your marketing plan, and 51 percent hard labor. So it comes down to valuing communication enough that PR will be given the basic marketing direction and people and that a budget will be assigned to get the job done.

The PR Disaster Plan

Sooner or later, disaster befalls almost any enterprise. A refinery blows up, a truck spills its cargo on the freeway, an officer of a bank embezzles $100,000, a store cashier is shot in a holdup, an airplane misses the runway, or a barge hits a bridge.

Sooner or later, something will happen at your hospital that will attract media attention. Precisely when the disaster strikes, just when everyone in the hospital is scrambling to sort out the problem, just when you can least afford the time, you will find every reporter and photographer in town at your door demanding answers and pictures.

That is why you need a carefully thought out public relations disaster plan. This plan should be put together by the PR staff, approved by the hospital management, and communicated with consummate care to department heads and anyone else in the hospital who might be on the receiving end of a reporter's call. All of this should happen a long time before a disaster hits.

The plan must anticipate the most likely emergencies and give specific instructions in plain, colloquial English, so that people under pressure can find answers in a hurry. The following passage includes the type of instructions that should appear in every hospital employee's procedures manual.

What to do if a reporter calls

1. Advise the reporter that you are not authorized to speak for the hospital. Tell the reporter you will transfer him or her to the proper person.

2. Transfer the reporter to Ms. Patricia Shrude in headquarters, at 641-9167. If Ms. Shrude cannot be reached, then proceed down this list of authorized company representatives:

   - Mr. Johnson on 641-9070
   - Ms. Zimmerman on 641-9171
   - And so on

3. Your job is to be helpful to the reporter and get him or her to the right person quickly; that's all. Be courteous and helpful, but do not answer questions or comments. Simply explain that you are not authorized to speak for the hospital.

Instructions to the top management persons, trustees, medical staff, and all department heads, will be more complete than that, but not much. The purpose is to get the reporter to the designated trained representatives.

These representatives will have a detailed set of instructions that will have been carefully worked out in advance. The instructions will be contained in a document titled "Hospital PR Disaster Plan: Instructions to Designated Representative" and will explain what to do if:

- There has been a fire
- A famous person enters or dies in the hospital
- A law suit is announced
- There is a major accident, and many people enter the hospital, and so on

In general, you will want to think through the ethical considerations for each event well in advance. And you will also have some legal considerations to think about.

The advantage of a carefully thought out PR disaster plan is that it allows the hospital to behave calmly and confidently in the middle of the storm. The hospital and its representative will usually emerge from the disaster, whatever it is, covered with raves if they have the plan ready to go when problems appear.

The Stress Interview:
Sweaty Palms Time

Much of the reluctance among hospital officials concerning public relations starts with the knowledge that there is a risk in granting interviews. Doctors are afraid that they will appear nonprofessional, and CEOs are aware that they can be embarrassed in front of the board of trustees or their peers at other hospitals. Trustees are equally leery of interviews. Sweaty palms time for most of us.

Often, hospital officials unwittingly opt for the course of action with the highest risk: avoiding the press altogether or clamming up and stonewalling it. The nagging worry that "I'll blow it" is widespread in our industry.

The quickest way I know to get over the worry and gain the confidence that you need in order to get in front of a camera, or even to answer the reporter's phone call, is to study the rudiments of successful interviewing and then rehearse and practice. Recognizing this, several organizations in the country offer programs for corporate executives (who all have lapses of confidence) on how to deal effectively with reporters.

When the cameras are rolling and the microphone is on, you are in a stress interview. Typical thoughts that run through your mind as the microphone is pushed in your face are "I won't get a second chance," "I have to look bright," "My friends will laugh," "What if my boss sees this?," and "What if they bring up that nasty mess we were in three years ago?"

As a survivor of an interview with Mike Wallace, I can assure you that you, too, can handle the tough interview. I was working for a retail firm, and one day, as I arrived at work, there was Mike Wallace on the telephone wanting to come and see me in one hour—with crew, with lights, and with equipment. What do you do? Do you say, "Yes," "No," "No comment," or what?

I took the safest route and said, "Let me do a little checking, and I'll get back." After a quick consultation with the president of the firm, I called back and told Mike Wallace to come ahead. My feeling was that there was risk to the company no matter what we did. But we had the least risk if we opened up and talked. The company was a totally honest enterprise, an admired member of the local business community with nothing to hide and plenty to be proud of. So we talked to *60 Minutes.*

An interview that lasted three hours showed up as a 90-second segment on the broadcast. CBS completed its story, and the company emerged unscathed with its reputation unblemished. And that is what it is all about.

At this particular company, the Mike Wallace interview led to training about 20 other executives in a course so that they were equipped for future experiences of this kind. What they did was to work their heads off, get miserably embarrassed, and completely blow interview after interview. But they made their mistakes in private. Finally, three days later, they emerged humbled but confident that they could handle about anything that came along.

You should consider such practice sessions for the top brass of your hospital, including the chairman of the board and the representatives for the medical staff. Learning to handle stressful interviews is part of the job in a hospital that is organizing for good PR.

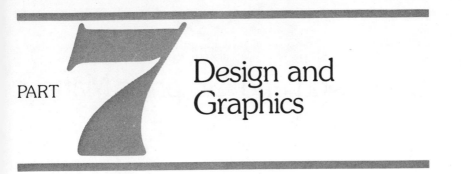

PART **7** Design and Graphics

Do Design and Graphics Matter?

Elements of a Graphic Design System

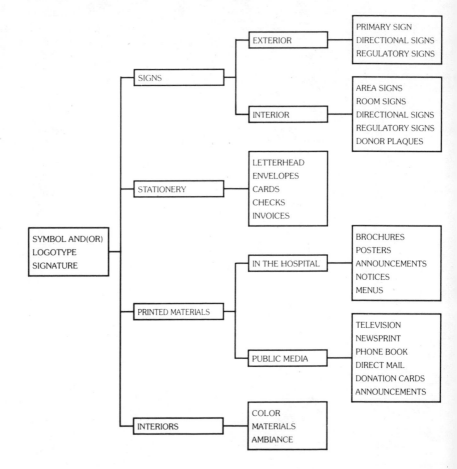

In a hospital, where great personal joys as well as considerable personal tragedies are experienced every day, does the absence of good graphics or design really make much difference? Does a consistent use of the "house" colors or the presence of good visual cues matter? Are such concerns extraneous or frivolous?

Our conviction is that they do indeed matter. They create moods, agreeable or disagreeable, for the staff. Design sets up expectations for patients and visitors. The design system is part of the environment of getting well, or perhaps even part of staying sick. So design and graphics are important.

The face that the hospital presents to the public is far more influential than is generally understood. Organizing graphics and putting design to work to express the hospital's mission statement and market positioning is one of the earliest marketing needs the hospital should address.

The chart on the previous page presents the items encompassed by the hospital's graphic design system. It shows how design begins with a corporate logotype and signature system and then spreads to all of the other communication vehicles of the hospital.

Finding the Right Designer and Establishing Rapport

Hiring a designer is not as easy as looking in the *Yellow Pages*. Designers are not all equal, and they are not all equally qualified for the job you want to get done. The purpose of this chapter is to give you some help in identifying the right designer for you and your hospital.

First, you should look for an *industrial* designer, someone who is able to work with and direct other specialists. The industrial designer is good at graphics, good at color, good at solving problems, good at using design as the vehicle. That covers a lot of ground, including interior design, design of special furniture, and so forth.

When you go shopping for the design firm, here are the things to look for:

1. *Hospital experience.* This may be the most important criterion. The designer should have experience with hospitals. Find one who has produced the whole graphics system for hospitals. Hospitals have some problems that are unique and tough to solve.
2. *Problem-solving ability.* Many designers are not oriented to problem solving; they are into the artsy-craftsy side, but they get hung up in their own priorities and forget what you are trying to accomplish. It is a good sign when the design firm you are interviewing asks, "What are you trying to do?" or "What does this institution stand for?" or "What is your strategy?"
3. *Ability to listen.* If the designer appears to listen well, to be intent on hearing you, that's good. If he wants to interview other people at the hospital, too, that is an even better sign.
4. *Discipline and implementation.* Does the designer exhibit a dogged determination to see his work fully implemented by his clients? Or is he content when the design is completed and presented? The clue here is this: when he was presenting his wares, did he show you the system you would use to make the program work?
5. *Respect for your assignment.* This is subjective, but you want someone working for you who thinks the job is important to him as well as to you. If he talks too much about giant jobs that he has

completed at 10 times the budget, you may be getting a clue that your assignment is beneath his dignity.

6. *Business skills.* Call some people who have worked with the designer before you hire him. Ask two questions: Did he bring the project to a conclusion, staying within the agreed-to-budget? Did he complete assignments on time? The main thing you should get from looking at the designer's previous work, however, is a sense that he has been solving problems, not just making pretty designs.

7. *Rapport.* You are going to live together for some months. Count on it—there will be some conflict and tension. Can you live together? If you doubt it up front, you are headed for disaster. Find someone you feel positive about. You should have fun working with a good designer. Keep looking until you get that feeling.

8. *Budget.* Money is always important (more about this in the next chapter).

9. *Previous assignments.* Did you like what you saw when you looked at previous work? You may not be a good judge of design, but you should have a feeling of respect for the work. Even better if your reaction was "Wow, that's great!"

Budgeting for Design Work

Budgeting for design is tricky because almost the same effort will go into a project for a 100-bed hospital as a 500-bed hospital. Partly, it is difficult because it is not repetitive. You don't do it every year. Typically, you need to budget for a big lump of work in the first year, followed by lesser amounts of continuing work in subsequent years. If done well, the basic core design work should last for several years.

Having said it is difficult, here is a starting place for you. Figure about 0.2 percent of the hospital's annual budget. That may not be enough for any size hospital, but it is a pretty good place to begin, and this is how that budget works out for hospitals of different sizes.

Total Annual Hospital Budget	Annual Design and Graphics Budget—0.2%
$ 5,000,000	$ 10,000
$10,000,000	$ 20,000
$20,000,000	$ 40,000
$50,000,000	$100,000

Over a five-year period, you will not spend the budget in neat increments. You are more likely to spend a five-year graphics and design budget by spending a big chunk in the first two years and then spending much less for the next three years. A hospital with a $10 million annual budget could appropriately budget to spend its total five-year design and graphic budget in the following increments:

Five-Year Design and Graphics Budget of a Hospital with a $10 Million Annual Budget

Year	Expenditure
1	$40,000
2	$30,000
3	$10,000
4	$10,000
5	$10,000

Achieving Effective Execution

The design scheme you use at your hospital should accurately reflect the mission statement of the hospital's long-range plan; it should be the visual expression of the hospital's market positioning.

Mere attractive design is relatively easy to achieve. Attractive design that expresses the hospital's direction is a much tougher assignment. But toughest of all is creating a consistency within the hospital and a design that is acceptable to the many people in managerial positions in the hospital. That is the only way the hospital can successfully express itself through the range of signs, forms, letterheads, and so on that it uses. That is tough.

You need not only good design, but also a system that locks the symbols and graphics into place so that you get performance. System means discipline; it means rules, a set of dos and don'ts. Free design counsel is often offered by forms suppliers, printers, and sign companies. The chances are good that the number of advertisers the hospital has used over the years is the main reason that it has deficiencies in the design area. You need to sort out and unify every single visual signal that your hospital sends out so that the signals say the same thing and create one single identity.

This is hard to achieve, simply because so many people in hospitals do not appreciate the importance of consistency, or they fail to recognize that the embellishments that they make subtract, rather than add, to the result. A hospital's design program must result in a graphics control document if you are to get effective execution.

Examples of Graphics Standards

Each hospital, just like each business enterprise, has its own graphics problems. And the need for a strong graphics system is just as important in a small hospital as it is in a large one.

Developing a graphics system is only half the battle; the other half is packaging the program so that the hospital can implement it after the designer has completed the project. To accomplish this, a graphics manual that specifies standards for the implementation of the design system is developed. Every issue is addressed, and nothing is left to chance. The following pages present design solutions for three Minnesota health care facilities: St. Louis Park Medical Center, an outpatient clinic located in St. Louis Park; Methodist Hospital, a 461-bed hospital in Minneapolis; and Queen of Peace Hospital, a 60-bed facility in New Prague.*

The selections of sample graphics standards presented here include a sample logotype and instructions for the use of a trademark (St. Louis Park Medical Center); trademark signatures and instructions for use of the trademark signatures and color specifications (Methodist Hospital); a letterhead design, instructions for letters and letterheads, sample booklets, and guidelines for the design of patient, community, and employee information booklets (Queen of Peace Hospital); and typography guidelines (St. Louis Park Medical Center).

---

*Artwork in this chapter provided courtesy of Ted Peterson Associates, Hinsdale, Illinois.

Organization/Identity Standards

The basic purpose of this manual is to introduce the new approved system for all visual communications. Outlined are the general guidelines for its use.

The guidelines, instructions, and reproduction materials available are to be used as aids in planning and executing our program effectively.

Our new program was developed in part to create a distinctive, contemporary, "family look" for the visual communications of the medical center, its foundations, divisions, and interests.

Once this is achieved, each form of communication will relate to and enforce every other.

Effective use of the trademark as an identifying device depends on accurate and controlled application. Only the reproduction art provided with this manual should be used for reproduction. The trademark may be enlarged or reduced photomechanically, as necessary. However, it should not be redrawn or traced, nor should the size and spacing relationships be altered, as any small variation in the design will change its character.

In all cases, it is imperative that the trademark be reproduced in accordance with procedures established in this manual. Persons dealing with suppliers who reproduce the trademark should insure that each supplier has a continuing supply of reproduction art. He should also insure that each supplier is well briefed on the guidelines pertaining to its use.

When preparing final art for those materials illustrated in this book, the size and position of the logotype, symbol, and typography are to be exactly as shown. Measurements should be taken directly from these pages. All typesetting is to follow the specifications. Layouts and keylines are to be submitted to the Department of Administration for approval prior to print.

Any questions regarding usage not covered by this guide may be referred to the Department of Administration, St. Louis Park Medical Center.

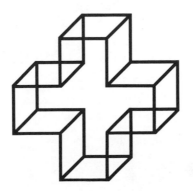

Methodist Hospital

6500 Excelsior Boulevard
St. Louis Park, Minnesota 55426
Telephone (612) 932-5000

Methodist Hospital Foundation

6500 Excelsior Boulevard
St. Louis Park, Minnesota 55426
Telephone (612) 932-5023

Methodist Hospital Auxiliary

6500 Excelsior Boulevard
St. Louis Park, Minnesota 55426
Telephone (612) 932-5000

Trademark Signatures and Color Specifications

Centered Version/Solid*
Shown are the recommended signatures for Methodist Hospital and its divisions.

The centered version should be used as the standard unless impractical because of space or layout requirements.

When address lines are used in print communications, they must be positioned as shown in the enlarged examples, using a Century Schoolbook typeface, no larger than 8 pt. with 1/2 pt. leading.

Color Specifications
The standard colors chosen for the Methodist Hospital and all of its divisions are: PMS 137 (marigold) and PMS 280 (blue).

The heart symbol should appear in PMS 137 (marigold) and the Methodist Hospital logotype and support copy should appear in PMS 280 (blue).

When printing in one color, other than black, both the symbol and logotype should appear in solid PMS 280 (blue).

When only black is available for printing, both symbol and logotype should appear in solid black. No screen tints should be used.

In special cases, the symbol and logotype may appear in white, reversed out of solid PMS 280 (blue) or black.

* The outline version of the symbol is available through the director of public relations.

301 Second Street, North East
New Prague, Minnesota 56071
(612) 758-4431
Metro: (612) 445-6530

Queen of Peace Hospital

July 24, 1981

Mr. John Doe
John Doe Associates
4616 N. Magnolia
Chicago, Illinois 60640

Dear John:

I believe that everything has been done in preparation for our meeting next week with the sign contractor. I have notified the personnel you requested to be in attendance, and all of them have the information that they need.

Should you have any further information or comments concerning our meeting, please be sure to let me know. I look forward to meeting with you on the 30th and will call you prior to that time to confirm your arrangements.

Sincerely,

Mary Smith
Community Relations

MS/fs

Stationery Guidelines:
Letterhead

This illustration shows the accepted version of a one-page letterhead.

All typewritten material should appear in a flush-left format. This means the left margin of all elements of the letter should align with the left edge of the printed address copy. Paragraphs are not indented.

Typewritten information should be positioned as shown, and should never appear crowded on the page. No line should be longer than 5½ " in order to maintain a right margin of 1½ ". The last entry on a given page should appear a minimum of 1" from the bottom of the page.

Printing Specifications

Stock:	Neenah/Classic Crest Avon Brilliant White 24 lb.—Wove Finish
Size:	8½ " x 11 "
Color:	Dove Symbol-PMS 343 (green) Logo and Address-PMS 409 (grey)
Typography:	Logo-14 pt. Times Bold Roman Address-7/7½ pt. Times Roman

Important Patient Information

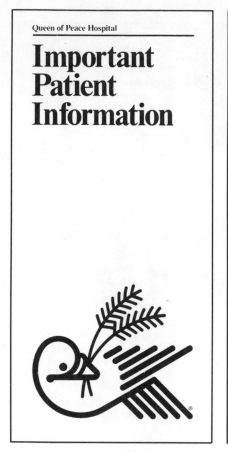

Parenthood Classes

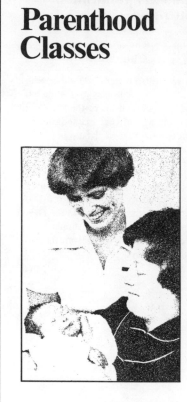

This example is used primarily for the presentation of important hospital policy or community information that requires a high level of hospital identification.

This example is used primarily for the presentation and explanation of general hospital services and procedures.

Informational Booklets:
Cover Formats

Queen of Peace Hospital

The Glucose Tolerance Test

How is one to assess and evaluate a type face in esthetic design? Why do pacemakers in the art rave over any specific face of type? Why is it so superlatively pleasant to their eyes? see in a good type design is. partly. its excellent fitness to perform its work. of its parts just right for its size. as any good tool good chair has all of its parts made nicely to the to do exactly the work that

How is one to assess and evaluate a type esthetic design? Why do pacemakers in the art of rave over any specific face of type? What do they Why is it so superlatively pleasant to their eyes? see in a good type design is. partly. its excellent fitness to perform its work. of its parts just right for its size. as any good tool good chair has all of its parts made nicely to the to do exactly the work that the chair has to do.

How is one to assess and evaluate a type face in esthetic design? Why do pacemakers in the art rave over any specific face of type? What do they Why is it so superlatively pleasant to their eyes? see in a good type design is. partly. its excellent fitness to perform its work. of its parts just right for its size. as any good tool good chair has all of its parts made nicely to the to do exactly the work that the chair

How is one to assess and evaluate a type face esthetic design? Why do pacemakers in the art rave over any specific face of type?

This example is used primarily for small amounts of information dealing with specific areas of medical care, such as outpatient care suggestions or specific procedures.

The illustrations shown are to be used for all general patient, community, and employee information booklets.

These different covers are used to distinguish or give emphasis to different levels of information. A general description is provided under each example.

Printing Specifications

Stocks: Champion/Kromekote CC2S Cover White/.010 (other Kromekote color stocks are optional.) Neenah/Classic Crest Grey 65 lb. Wove Finish (other Classic Crest Wove Finish color stocks are optional.)

One-Color: Dove symbol and all other information should appear in solid PMS 409 (grey), or black. When photography is used all materials should appear in a black halftone or mezzotint.

Two-Color: Dove symbol, headings and rule lines appear in PMS 343 (green) Logotype, address copy, and all other information appears in PMS 409 (grey) or black. When photography is used, regular halftones or mezzotint halftones may appear in either PMS 409 (grey) or black.

Typography Guidelines

Friz Quadrata is the established typeface to be used for all primary and divisional signature applications.

Friz Quadrata Bold may be used only in situations where special emphasis is necessary.

Helvetica is the established typeface to be used for all secondary information. Helvetica Regular is to be used for all brochure text, captions, address lines, and so on.

Helvetica Medium may be used wherever special emphasis is necessary (headlines, subheads, and so on).

Since there are slight variations in established typefaces, depending on where the type is purchased, special care must be taken to match exactly the letterforms displayed.

Friz Quadrata Bold

**ABCDEFGHIJKLMNOPQRSTUVWXYZ
abcdefghijklmnopqrstuvwxyz
$1234567890**

Friz Quadrata

ABCDEFGHIJKLMNOPQRSTUVWXYZ
abcdefghijklmnopqrstuvwxyz
$1234567890

Helvetica Medium

**ABCDEFGHIJKLMNOPQRSTUVWXYZ
abcdefghijklmnopqrstuvwxyz
$1234567890**

Helvetica Regular

ABCDEFGHIJKLMNOPQRSTUVWXYZ
abcdefghijklmnopqrstuvwxyz
$1234567890

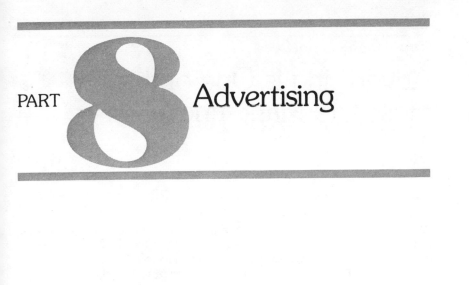

PART **8** Advertising

Advertising Is One of the Hospital's Marketing Tools

A couple of years ago, the public relations director of a large Eastern medical center asked me, "Should hospitals advertise?" My answer was yes. However, I would qualify that yes to say that hospitals must use this marketing technique not like amateurs, but with the same care that the professionals lavish on it.

Advertising is not an exact science; it is an art form. It can be used with great effectiveness or with indifferent results. It is an art form that has been experimented with over a great many years, and there are some real techniques to be applied.

I think advertising has survived as a marketing tool of the business community for one reason: it has been proven 10,000 times over to be legitimate, effective, and cost efficient.

Advertising is a legitimate tool of any enterprise that has honest communication needs to serve. There are many times when public relations tools are to be preferred. However, there are times when communication needs are better served by advertising. For one thing, advertising has the great virtue of being totally controllable by the advertiser. In addition, it has the great virtue of being cheap to use. For instance, many hospitals now routinely publish their annual reports as an advertisement. Just a few years ago, this was considered a daring innovation. The reason many now use newspapers for this purpose is that they recognize they can reach more people at lower cost than they could with the annual report that was mailed out.

Effective advertising is almost always the consequence of orderly, systematic, and logical thinking through of problems. Good advertising generally is the result of a sequence of events.

The hospital must first figure out its problems. It must absolutely understand whom it is willing to not reach. Generally, that means good marketing research is needed. The hospital also must figure out its present positioning—what it stands for and what it wants to stand for. (*Positioning* is marketing's word for the planner's word *mission*.) After having figured out what your problems are, what you stand for, whom you want to reach, you must figure out what your message is.

Now you are ready to consider whether you want to use advertising at all. It is entirely possible that the best answer to your problem is a private conversation with someone in the hallway. That's one way to get a job done. On the other hand, you might figure that advertising is indeed the right answer.

After having decided that advertising fits your needs, and you have a message that can best be conveyed through advertising, you can ask what medium you should use: newspapers, magazines, direct mail, television, radio, or something else?

This sequence is, of course, the ABCs of advertising, and it may sound a little insulting. In your discussions with doctors and administrators, you will generally find that the reaction to the use of advertising ranges from apathetic (the most positive end of the spectrum) to violently negative. You will hear most of them say things such as, "It isn't done," "It is so unseemly," "It's unprofessional," and so on.

Many thoughtful people disagree with this rather elitist view and consider it outdated. At all times, the medical profession and the health care industry are obligated to do two things: communicate with the people who are entitled to know what is going on in your hospital or in the health care system, and communicate at the lowest possible cost. Often, that means using advertising.

That's the case for advertising by hospitals. But that is *not* the case for all hospitals and probably not for any one hospital all the time. The argument is simply that when the time comes for you to use advertising, go to it. Do it professionally, and do it carefully. But don't hang back because "it isn't done" or it is "unprofessional." Advertising is a good, sturdy, and reliable tool for use by the hospital *when needed*.

Does Advertising Cost Too Much?

"It costs too much" is the reaction of many administrators and trustees to the idea of using advertising. "All we can afford are postcards" is the way it is frequently stated. Actually, if you wish to reach a broad audience of consumers, the mass media may be more economical. An examination of the cost of advertising using the postcard as a reference point is in order.

Medium	Cost per Message to Reach One Adult*
Postcard	$0.13
Half-page newspaper ad	$0.008
Full-page consumer magazine	$0.009
30-second prime-time TV spot	$0.005
30-second TV local spot	$0.007

Although the foregoing comparison of media costs is a crude one, it demonstrates the reason businesses use mass media rather than post-cards when they need to communicate with consumers in large num-bers. Businessmen believe they have an obligation to their stockhold-ers to use the most efficient media available. Can hospitals do less? It would seem self-evident that they cannot.

However, this raises another issue. How much advertising does it take to *register* the message? Most persons underestimate how much effort it takes because they assume that if they publish their advertise-ment in the newspaper, just about everyone will get the message and remember it. Registering the message is not that simple.

Assume that a population of 1,000 persons is to be reached and that you will use a one-half page newspaper advertisement. Here is what

*Data in the chapter were provided by N. W. Ayer Incorporated, New York City.

will happen if the advertisement is very good and gets better than average attention and readership.

	Percent	Number of Persons
Starting population	100%	1,000
Population minus percentage of population who does not read newspaper on typical day (varies by market)	50%	500
Population minus percentage of readers (15%) who do not look at any given page	43%	425
Population minus percentage of readers who do not read any given ad (75%)	11%	106

Thus from a base of 1,000 persons, the advertisement actually reached only 11%—or 106 people. That is a loss of 89%—or 894 consumers—the advertisement was intended to reach. Now build in the fact that no one recalls everything he has read or learned, and a month or so later perhaps a couple of dozen of the 106 persons of the original 1,000 base will remember the advertisement.

This explains why experienced advertisers use campaigns instead of single ads when they need to reach a large number of persons. You need to think about a series of messages, or the same message repeated many times, if you hope to reach a significant portion, say 50 percent, of your audience. It takes a lot of effort to reach out and get the message to a large audience. There are no free lunches, and you must realize this when you begin budgeting for advertising.

Selecting Your Audience and the Medium to Fit

In the previous chapter, it was assumed that you want to reach a broad audience of consumers, but often that will not be the case. Therefore, on many occasions, the broad-reach media (newspapers, TV, radio) may not be the preferred ones to use for your hospital's message.

Before the medium is selected or a piece of copy is written, you must answer an important question: whom is the hospital trying to reach? In hospital marketing, there are four likely target audiences:

1. The doctors who practice at your hospital and sometimes the other doctors in the community
2. The hospital family—that is, everyone who is associated with the hospital
3. Members of the health systems agency and other regulatory health agencies and politicians
4. A broad consumer audience

Once the audiences are defined, the spectrum of media available is probably a little bigger than you think. It includes:

* Personal visits
* Phone calls and personal letters
* Preprinted postcards and letters
* Printed brochures mailed to individuals
* Printed brochures mass-mailed to homes in a selected area (around your hospital, for instance)
* Magazines (city or metropolitan editions)
* Radio (selected specific audiences, based on the kind of program format)
* Newspapers (to reach adult audiences)
* Billboards
* Television

The media are arranged from the most specific, most personal, and most expensive to the most "mass" and the cheapest on a *cost per exposure basis.* Which you will use depends to a considerable degree on the audience you are trying to reach and influence. It also depends on what your message is.

For instance, you might want to reach a group of city council members or 100 state legislators. On the basis of audience information only, you might elect to write each individual a series of letters. However, recognizing the political nature of the audiences just identified, the hospital might on certain occasions prefer to reach them through a full-page newspaper advertisement. That way the audience will get the message, but so will the voters, to whom your audience is accountable. Remember that what determines the medium isn't just the message or just the audience. Usually it is both.

If your hospital is in a small town, you often must look for doctors to locate in your community. If you knew where those doctors were, you could write to them. But you don't know, so you go to another medium, such as magazines. For instance, you advertise in a special-audience magazine like *Country Journal,* because you recognize that some of its readers are doctors who live in big cities but who would prefer to live in a small town. Or you advertise in a hunting and fishing magazine for the same reason. Some of its readers will be doctors who yearn for a practice closer to the fishing.

The audience you want to reach plus the message you want to deliver will usually be the main determinants of the media you use. Media selection is not as obvious as you might at first believe. You need to think about it and work at it. You may want to hire an advertising agency to help you.

The Leverage Is in the Message

You can't do a lot to change the cost of a newspaper page, but you can dramatically increase (or decrease) the number of persons you can reach by the interest you create in your message. Some advertisers get 8 or 10 times the number of readers that others do, using the same unit job space or time. The reason is that some advertisers are simply more effective in expressing themselves. Some are more creative and write more interesting advertisements. Some know how to use the media, and some don't.

This is why you shouldn't have committees of trustees, or lawyers, or administrators attempting to write the ads. The result is predictable—an advertisement that, although factually accurate and legally correct, almost no one will read.

Copy writing is a high-quality craft to which you should pay attention. Buying the space or time at the right price is easy compared to putting your message into the right combination of words and pictures so that it registers in the heads of a large proportion of the hospital's audience. Getting those people to act on the information is what you are after.

The message is: get the very best professional you can afford to develop your advertising. The skilled professional cannot change the cost of the space or time, but he can cut the *cost per person reached* by 80 or 90 percent by reaching eight or nine times more people than a less skilled professional would. Dull advertisements cost as much as creative, interesting advertisements, but the interesting advertisements are read by 8 or 10 times more people.

9

The Marketing Budget and the Marketing Audit

The Marketing Budget: A Beginning Point

In the end, your convictions about marketing will be tested by how much money you are willing to allocate to the effort. Likewise, your belief that consumers' opinions and attitudes are important to your hospital will be tested and measured by the dollars you invest in consumer research. Finally, just how serious you are about communicating will be reflected in the budget that is finally approved by the board for such line items as public relations, graphics and design, and advertising.

Nevertheless, you need a starting point for your budget, and this is it. Following are the values I place on the various functions we have discussed. When you add them all up, you have the basis for the total marketing budget.

Activity	Percent of Hospital's Total Budget to be Allocated	Priority	Comments
Marketing planning and marketing audit	0.1%	1	This is the cost of the original planning and organizing of the marketing effort, plus an annual review to upgrade the program for better results.
Consumer research	0.5%	1	This is the cost of listening, which provides the basis for the hospital's long-range planning effort as well as its marketing effort.
Design and graphics	0.2%	2	Creation of a solid graphics system is given the second priority because it is an area where marketing can make an immediate impact.

| Public relations and advertising | 0.7% | 2 | Public relations and advertising are given second priority as well, second behind consumer research and planning, because the hospital will emerge with a stronger communications program if it is based on research and expresses a complete marketing plan. |
| | | | Note that the split between advertising and PR will vary among hospitals and over time. |

When you take these percentages and apply them to hospitals of various sizes, here are the marketing budgets you arrive at. These budgets assume a maturity that probably does not exist in your hospital as you begin your marketing effort.

Mature Marketing Budgets

Hospital Budget	Planning and Audit 0.1%	Market Research 0.5%	Design and Graphics 0.2%	PR and Advertising 0.7%	Total 1.5%
$ 5 million	$ 5,000	$ 25,000	$ 10,000	$ 35,000	$ 75,000
$10 million	$10,000	$ 50,000	$ 20,000	$ 70,000	$150,000
$20 million	$20,000	$100,000	$ 40,000	$140,000	$300,000
$50 million	$50,000	$250,000	$100,000	$350,000	$750,000

Next, you need to consider the probable sequence of events. Assuming that your hospital has little marketing activity at present, an annual hospital budget of $10 million, and an 8 percent annual inflation rate, here is how you would expect the budget to grow from year 1.

Beginning Four-Year Marketing Budget
for Hospital with $10 Million Annual Budget

Year	Hospital Budget— $ Millions	Planning and Audit	Market Research	Design and Graphics	PR and Advertising	Total Marketing
1	10.0	$25,000	$50,000	—	—	$ 75,000
2	10.8	$10,800	$54,000	$40,000	$ 70,000	$174,800
3	11.7	$11,700	$58,500	$30,000	$ 75,300	$175,500
4	12.6	$12,600	$63,000	$10,000	$103,400	$189,000

As you see, the budget builds through a sequence like that shown above, with start-up costs reflected in planning and market research. Later expenditures for graphics, PR, and advertising reflect the orderly addition of new marketing functions. So a hospital that is starting from scratch, with no budget, no staff, and no experience, does not launch into a full-blown program in the first year.

This is the beginning point for your own thinking about the costs of marketing. Only you can decide on the value your hospital can gain through these expenditures. Only you can assess the costs of *not* getting into marketing at your hospital.

The Marketing Audit: Getting It Right

Very few effective marketing efforts are created from whole cloth. Most undergo steady change. The hospital's long-range plan and its basic market positioning are bedrocks, the solid foundation on which the marketing strategy rests. But priorities change, competition changes, the government's programs change, consumer needs and worries change. All of these make it natural and appropriate that the hospital change its marketing programs in response.

There is another reason you should expect change: you won't get it right the first time out. The best marketing people don't, and you should not expect to beat the odds. The very best plans in marketing frequently yield surprises. Effective marketing programs are generally the result of learning from and correcting a string of failures. So the trick is to keep trying, assess the results quickly, and make appropriate course corrections.

Your marketing effort should be examined at least yearly to be sure that it is still on target. Each part of the program should be examined in an annual audit and challenged—found appropriate or found wanting. The marketing audit takes the values that most commercial enterprises get from test marketing and translates them to the hospital setting. The marketing audit reflects the fact that hospitals are different from other marketers, but still have the need to challenge their programs and learn from the mistakes.

The marketing audit is one way by which hospitals are going to get good at the job. In five years the leading hospitals will be using marketing techniques effectively and routinely. An annual examination—probably by an outsider with perspective and experience and working with a small team from the senior administrative staff and a few board members—will be one of the key tools used to ensure that progress is being made.

Marketing is a tool of the hospital's aspirations. The marketing audit should ensure that marketing accurately expresses the long-range strategy and helps to implement the strategy through appropriate and steadily improving use of marketing techniques.

A Sample Marketing Assessment/Audit

What follows is a marketing assessment, or audit. This questionnaire is to be filled out by a CEO, or his/her designee. Its intent is to elicit some preliminary information and also to get some thinking started.

Respondents are asked to fill out the questionnaire as completely as possible, but not to worry if there are questions that cannot be responded to at the time.

1. **Marketing Decision-Making Apparatus**

   A. Who in the hospital do you think will set the hospital's marketing strategy and make the big decisions?

      The CEO? _____

      A board committee? _____

      A vice-president of marketing? _____

      Other? Please describe. _____

      _____

   B. Who in the hospital do you expect to be the main initiators of marketing actions?

      The CEO? _____

      A board committee? _____

      A vice-president of marketing? _____

      Someone else in the community? _____

      Who? _____

      The HSA? _____

      Other? Please describe. _____

   C. Who else do you expect to participate in the hospital's marketing decision-making process? Please describe.

      _____

2. Use of Outside Consultants vs. Doing the Work In-House

Marketing is generally thought to encompass a number of specialist areas, listed below. Please indicate which of these activities you would expect to do in-house and those services you would expect to hire from outside the organization.

Marketing Specialty	In-House Activity	Service Hired Outside
Development of marketing strategy	_____	_____
Marketing management	_____	_____
Research of consumer attitudes about our hospital	_____	_____
Research of physician attitudes about our hospital	_____	_____
Public relations	_____	_____
Internal publications	_____	_____
Design and graphics	_____	_____
Advertising	_____	_____

3. Priorities

Question 2 listed the activities that are generally thought to be part of marketing. Here is the same list. Please indicate the areas for which you feel the greatest sense of urgency. Do this by placing the number 1 after the activity of greatest urgency, 2 after the item of next greatest urgency, and so forth.

Development of marketing strategy _____

Marketing management _____

Research of consumer attitudes about our hospital _____

Research of physician attitudes about our hospital _____

Public relations _____

Internal publications _____

Design and graphics _____

Advertising _____

4. Making Things Happen

Once the decisions are made, whom do you expect to be involved, on an ongoing basis, with implementing the decisions—making things happen? Some possibilities are listed below. Please indicate how you see them being employed.

A. The hospital's public relations department _____

_____

B. The administrative staff _____

_____

C. A marketing manager hired from outside _____

_____

D. Volunteers _____

_____

E. An outside consumer research firm _____

_____

F. An outside public relations firm _____

_____

G. An outside advertising agency _____

_____

H. Others. What other thoughts do you have? _____

_____

_____

5. Budget

What budget do you see being made available for marketing activities over the next five years?

	$XXX
Year 1	_____
Year 2	_____
Year 3	_____
Year 4	_____
Year 5	_____

6. **Sources of Information**

  A. Although marketing techniques have been used extensively by business for many years, they have not been widely used by hospitals. How did you first hear about marketing?

    _____

    _____

    _____

  B. How do you expect to keep abreast of the marketing field?

    _____

    _____

    _____

7. **Issues and Objectives**

With what issues at your hospital do you expect marketing to be most helpful?

  Issue 1. _____

    _____

    _____

  Issue 2. _____

    _____

    _____

  Issue 3. _____

    _____

    _____

What objectives will you set for the marketing activities of your hospital?

  1. _____

  2. _____

  3. _____

8. **Mission and Long-Range Plan**

Marketing should serve the needs of the hospital's long-range plan. It should express the hospital's mission statement and make it "live." Please attach the hospital's

- Mission statement
- Long-range plan

9. **Data**

A. Please describe or, if possible, attach any consumer research done for the hospital.

   _____

   _____

B. Please describe, or attach, any data you have about physicians' attitudes toward the hospital.

   _____

   _____

C. Please describe, or attach, any consumer research done to compare this hospital with alternative consumer choices, such as health maintenance organizations, surgery centers, and so on.

   _____

   _____

D. Please describe, or attach, any studies done by government agencies that might be pertinent to your marketing effort.

   _____

   _____

E. Please attach a map of the hospital showing its location and the location of competitive hospitals or alternative sources of treatment.

F. Please attach a list of each of your competitors showing
   - Total number of beds in use
   - Number of beds assigned to each department
   - Percentage utilization of each department for past five years

G. Please attach an assortment of the hospital's internal forms.

H. Please attach a complete package of any forms, letters, letterheads, brochures, or pamphlets that patients have seen in the past 12 months.

I. Please enclose snapshots or slides showing the hospital's interior and exterior signs.

J. Please enclose any advertising that your hospital has placed in the media (like newspapers) in the past three years. (If broadcast media were used, enclose the scripts.)

K. Please enclose "clips" of any articles about your hospital that have appeared in the past year.

10. Other

A. In your opinion, what data should be asked for? Please list.

_____

_____

_____

_____

B. What other questions should have been asked? Please write them down.

_____

_____

_____

C. Which 'questions need re-working to make them easier to understand and respond to?

_____

_____

_____

Filling the Marketing Director's Job

You should now be ready to ask these questions: Who should lead this marketing effort? Should we bring in an outside marketing "expert" and teach this person something about hospitals? Should we take one of the administrative staff and get this person to learn marketing?

The argument in favor of the experienced hospital administrator is that he knows how to get along in the hospital environment and knows the ropes. He isn't likely to upset the doctors or ruffle the feathers of the trustees. A hospital is a complex organization, and it is easy for the outsider to stub his toe. Yet it may be faster for the marketing person to learn about the hospital than for the hospital administrator to learn the subtleties of marketing. The reason is that there is a lot of expertise in the hospital available at all times to help the marketing person learn. But there are no marketing people in the hospital to help hospital people avoid the many pitfalls of marketing. It is a tough choice.

Candidates with master of hospital administration (MHA) degrees have not usually had marketing experience, and marketing usually has not been dealt with in great depth in their education. Further, it is going to be a tough sell convincing a lot of young administrators that they should take a detour into marketing. It is not likely to be viewed as the fast track to the top.

There is a similar problem with bringing experienced marketing managers into the hospital. At the present time, hospitals may appear as the pony leagues of marketing—a dead end, not a place to sharpen your skills, not the big time. Five years from now, it seems likely that marketing will be big in the curriculum for MHAs, and hospitals may be one of the logical career steps for aspiring marketing people.

Meanwhile, the hospital attempting to fill the job of marketing director has three choices.

1. *Combine marketing with the planning function.* There is a logic to this because of the inherent overlap between the functions. This is the first choice, even though the majority of hospital planning direc-

tors have little experience in marketing and tend to underestimate the job. In spite of these problems, this will probably prove to be the right decision for most hospitals.

2. *Promote the hospital's public relations director.* This is a real possibility in hospitals that now employ high-powered public relations talent. For many hospitals, however, this isn't going to work. Marketing is not synonymous with public relations, and a long career in hospital PR work does not automatically mean that person can function as the marketing director.

3. *Hire a marketing professional.* The best candidate will be a seasoned professional who may have decided he wants a change of atmosphere.

So there are no pat answers.

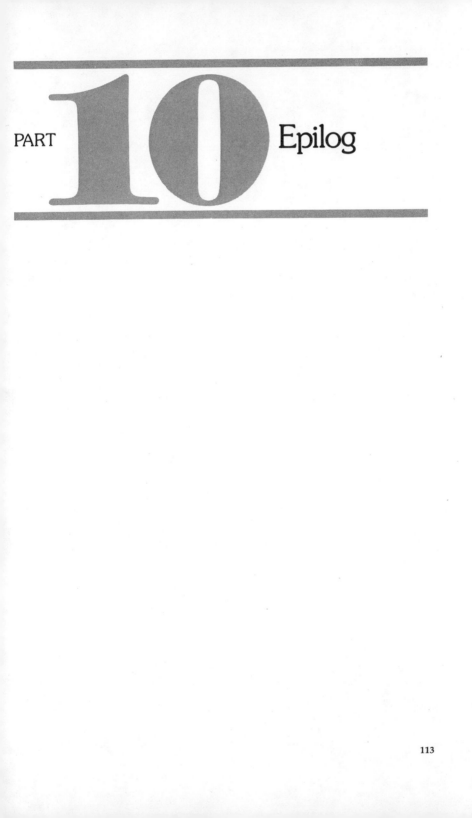

PART **10** Epilog

The Last Word

The basic premise of this book is a simple one: Hospitals need to get consumers into the act, get them involved in the key decisions being made about their hospitals, and this needs to be done now.

All through the '70s, society continued to register its displeasure with the system of health care. Elected officials responded by proposing new laws and regulations and making daily speeches that produced headlines and promised even more unpleasant news.

There is a more constructive alternative to this state of affairs, and that is to bring consumers into the act in a meaningful, productive way. There is a way to listen more intelligently, a way to hear with precision, a way to establish an early warning system so that hospitals can see problems in advance rather than constantly putting out fires. There is a way to enhance communication between hospitals and their constituencies through proven techniques that are available to everyone. Those techniques are ready for use, they work, they are not mysterious, and they are not costly.

All of this—the willingness to listen, the willingness to seek out and understand consumers' desires and anxieties, the willingness on the part of hospitals to communicate openly with society with trust and respect—the sum of those parts is an art form called marketing.

Bibliography

Anderson, D., and Kerr, M. Citizen influence in health service programs. In: Rosen, H. and others, editors. *The Consumer and the Health Care System*. New York City: Spectrum Publications, 1977.

Applebaum, A. Hospitals must be businesslike. *Hospitals, J.A.H.A.* 53:107, Oct. 1, 1979.

Behrens, R. Climate ripe for marketing strategies. *Hospitals, J.A.H.A.* 53:99, Oct. 1, 1979.

Berkowitz, E., and Flexner, W. The marketing audit: A tool for health service organizations. *Health Care Manage. Rev.* 3:51, Fall 1978.

Clarke, R. Marketing health care: Problems in implementation. *Health Care Manage. Rev.* 3:21, Winter 1978.

Clarke, R., and Sorey, H. The board's role in marketing the hospital. *Trustee.* 32:39, May 1979.

Cohn, V. Is the press telling the health story? In: Goodwin, I., editor. *Paying for American's Health Care*. Action, MA: Publishing Sciences Group, 1973.

Cooper, P. and Maxwell III, R. Marketing: Entry points and pitfalls. *Hosp. and Health Services Admin.* 24:34, Summer 1979.

Cunningham, R. Of snake oil and science. *Trustee.* 52:34, April 1978.

Dornblaser, B. The social responsibility of general hospitals. *Hosp. Admin.* 14:6, Spring 1969.

Echeveste, D. W., and Schlacter, J. L. Marketing a strategic framework for health care. *Nurs. Outlook.* 22:377, June 1974.

Effect of medical staff characteristics on hospital cost. *Soc. Security Bull.* 40:3, Dec. 1977.

Enthoven, A. Consumer-centered vs. job-centered health insurance. *Harvard Bus. Rev.* 57:141, Jan.-Feb. 1979.

Flexner, W., and others. Discovering what the health consumer really wants. *Health Care Manage. Rev.* 2:43, Fall 1977.

FTC judge: Doctors should be free to advertise. *Advertising Age.* 49: Dec. 9, 1978.

Geltzer, H. A marketing strategy for hospitals. *Hosp. Forum* 19:4, Dec. 1976.

Gregg, T., and Voyvodich, M. Marketing: Fast becoming a necessary tool for hospital administrators. *Hospitals, J.A.H.A.* 53:141, Apr. 1, 1979.

Griest, D. H. Choice is not whether, but rather how, to market health care institutions. *Hosp. Financial Manage.* 28:58, Jan. 1974.

Herzlingher, R. Can we control health care costs? *Harvard Bus. Rev.* 46:102, Mar.-Apr. 1978.

Hospital administration currents. *Ross Timesaver.* 23:1, Jan.-Feb. 1976. (Newsletter of Ross Laboratories, Columbus, OH)

Hunt, S. D. The nature and scope of marketing. *J. of Marketing.* 40:17, July 1976.

Ireland, R. Using marketing strategies to put hospitals on target. *Hospitals, J.A.H.A.* 51:54, June 1, 1977.

Johnson Jr., R. L. Going for broke: The hospital/government game. *Hosp. Financial Manage.* 31:9, Aug. 1977.

Kaplan, M. What it is, what it isn't. *Hospitals, J.A.H.A.* 53:176, Sept. 16, 1979.

Kotler, P. A generic concept of marketing. *J. of Marketing.* 36:46, Apr. 1972.

_____. *Marketing for Nonprofit Organizations.* Englewood Cliffs, NJ: Prentice-Hall, Inc., 1975.

Kurtz, H. P. *Public Relations and Fund Raising for Hospitals.* Springfield, IL: Charles C Thomas, 1980.

Lazer, W., and Kelley, E. J., editors. *Social Marketing: Perspectives and Viewpoints.* Homewood, IL: Richard D. Irwin, Inc., 1973.

Lindsey, H. T. Social auditing. *Hosp. Financial Manage.* 33:32, May 1979.

MacStravic, R. E. *Marketing Health Care.* Germantown, MD: Aspen Systems Corporation, 1977.

Neuhauser, D. The public voice and the nation's health. *Millbank Memorial Fund Quarterly* 57:60, Winter 1979.

O'Hallaron, R. D., and others. Marketing your hospital. *Hosp. Prog.* 57:68, Dec. 1976.

Palmer, M. Tell your story with ads. *Hosp. Financial Manage.* 32:50, Feb. 1978.

Riggs, F. Team PR. *Hosp. Financial Manage.* 33:12, May 1979.

Rummer, P. Public relations: Putting the cost puzzle together. *Hosp. Financial Manage.* 32:12, Jan. 1978.

Shapiro, B. P. *Marketing in Nonprofit Organizations.* Cambridge, Marketing Science Institute, 1972.

Simon, J. Marketing the community hospital: A tool for the beleagured administrator. *Health Care Manage. Rev.* 3:11, Spring 1978.

Smejda, H. How one hospital sells expertise to industry. *Hosp. Financial Manage.* 31:8, Oct. 1977.

Thieme, C. W., and others. Strategic planning has market orientation. *Hospitals, J.A.H.A.* 53:57, Dec. 1, 1979.

Tyson, T. Tyson: Hospitals need marketing help. *Advertising Age*. 49:6, Feb. 13, 1978.

Tucker, S. L. Introducing marketing as a planning and management tool. *Hosp. and Health Services Admin.* 22:37, Winter 1977.

Ziff, D. Community relations: Hospitals engage in educational marketing efforts. *Hospitals, J.A.H.A.* 52:69, Apr. 1, 1978.